Manipal Handbook on

Drugs, Contraceptives and Instruments in
Obstetrics and Gynecological Nursing

Manipal Handbook on

Drugs, Contraceptives and Instruments in Obstetrics and Gynecological Nursing

Faculty
Department of Obstetrics and Gynecological Nursing
Manipal College of Nursing
Manipal Academy of Higher Education
Manipal
Karnataka

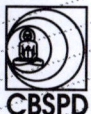

CBS Publishers & Distributors Pvt Ltd

New Delhi • Bengaluru • Chennai • Kochi • Kolkata • Lucknow • Mumbai
Hyderabad • Jharkhand • Nagpur • Patna • Pune • Uttarakhand

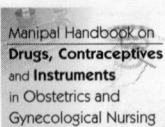

Manipal Handbook on
Drugs, Contraceptives
and **Instruments**
in Obstetrics and
Gynecological Nursing

ISBN: 978-93-877-4284-0

First Edition: 2018

Reprint: 2024

Published by Satish Kumar Jain and produced by Varun Jain for

CBS Publishers & Distributors Pvt Ltd

4819/XI Prahlad Street, 24 Ansari Road, Daryaganj, New Delhi 110 002, India.
Ph: 23289259, 23266861   Website: www.cbspd.com
                            e-mail: delhi@cbspd.com

Corporate Office: 204 FIE, Industrial Area, Patparganj, Delhi 110 092

Ph: 4934 4934   Fax: 4934 4935   e-mail: publishing@cbspd.com; publicity@cbspd.com

Branches

- **Bengaluru:** Seema House 2975, 17th Cross, K.R. Road,
  Banasankari 2nd Stage, Bengaluru 560 070, Karnataka
  Ph: +91-80-26771678/79   Fax: +91-80-26771680   e-mail: bangalore@cbspd.com

- **Chennai:** 7, Subbaraya Street, Shenoy Nagar, Chennai 600 030, Tamil Nadu
  Ph: +91-44-26680620, 26681266   Fax: +91-44-42032115   e-mail: chennai@cbspd.com

- **Kochi:** 42/1325, 1326, Power House Road, Opp KSEB, Ernakulam 682 018,
  Kochi, Kerala, India
  Ph: +91-484-4059061-65   Fax: +91-484-4059065   e-mail: kochi@cbspd.com

- **Kolkata:** 147, Hind Ceramics Compound, 1st Floor, Nilgunj Road, Belghoria,
  Kolkata 700 056, West Bengal, India
  Ph: +91-33-25633055/56   e-mail: kolkata@cbspd.com

- **Lucknow:** Basement, Khushnuma Complex, 7-Meerabai Marg
  (Behind Jawahar Bhawan), Lucknow 226 001, UP, India
  Ph: +0552-4000032   e-mail:tiwari.lucknowi@cbspd.com

- **Mumbai:** PWD Shed. Gala no. 25/26, Ramchandra Bhatt Marg, Next to JJ Hospital
  Gate no. 2, Opp. Union Bank of India, Noorbaug, Mumbai 400 009, Maharashtra, India
  Ph: 022-66661880/89   e-mail: mumbai@cbspd.com

Representatives

- **Hyderabad** 0-9885175004 • **Jharkhand** 0-9811541605 • **Nagpur** 0-8692091830
- **Patna** 0-9334159340 • **Pune** 0-9664372571 • **Uttarakhand** 0-9716462459

Printed at Chaman Enterprises, Daryaganj, Delhi, India

Preface

Manipal Handbook on Drugs, Contraceptives and Instruments in Obstetrics and Gynecological Nursing is comprehensive, logically organized, user-friendly and written in a very simple language for the understanding of the undergraduate nursing students. It offers the learners' a wide coverage of topics that are commonly included in obstetrics and gynecological nursing, which include instruments and the drugs most commonly used for obstetric and gynecological patients. The book also covers the family planning methods/contraceptives which will be beneficial for the practical preparedness of the students. The content is logically presented with simplified forms and terms that help the learners to understand and practice in the clinical area. Clear and brief description of content with proper figures and diagrams are provided for easy understanding of subject.

The authors are full-time teaching faculty, qualified with Master's degree in Nursing, of Department of obstetrics and Gynecological Nursing, Manipal College of Nursing, MAHE. The faculty are constantly involved in teaching, clinical services, and research.

Target Audience: This handbook has been written mainly for the undergraduate nursing students; it will also be useful to the diploma nursing and postgraduate nursing students for developing practical knowledge in obstetric and gynecological nursing for the preparation of practical examination. It can also be used as a bedside guide.

The manual primarily aims at the undergraduate and postgraduate students, and the midwives. It has evolved to provide comprehensive updated information in a concise and easy to read format. The chapters are extensively reviewed and organized following the recent guidelines from ACOG, WHO, NICE, and so on and also illustrated with figures and photographs.

Presentation of summary tables are special attraction which helps for easy comprehension and recapitulation.

We hope that this comprehensive book becomes an immense educational treasure for the readers.

Faculty
Department of Obstetrics and
Gynecological Nursing
MCON, Manipal, MAHE

Contributors

1. Drugs

Dr Judith Angelitta Noronha PhD, M Phil, MSc (N)
Professor and Associate Dean
Department of Obstetrics and Gynecological Nursing
Manipal College of Nursing, Manipal, MAHE

Dr Sushmitha Karkada PhD, MSc (N)
Assistant Professor
Department of Obstetrics and Gynecological Nursing
Manipal College of Nursing, Manipal, MAHE

Mrs Shobha MSc (N)
Lecturer
Department of Obstetrics and Gynecological Nursing
Manipal College of Nursing, Manipal, MAHE

2. Instruments

Dr Sonia RB D'Souza MA (Sociology), MSc (N), PhD
Associate Professor
Department of Obstetrics and Gynecological Nursing
Manipal College of Nursing, Manipal, MAHE

Mrs Pratibha Kamath MSc (N)
Assistant Professor
Department of Obstetrics and Gynecological Nursing
Manipal College of Nursing, Manipal, MAHE

3. Contraceptives

Dr Maria Pais MBA, PhD, MSc (N)
Assistant Professor
Department of Obstetrics and Gynecological Nursing
Manipal College of Nursing, Manipal, MAHE

Mrs Anusuya Prabhu MSc (N)
Assistant Professor
Department of Obstetrics and Gynecological Nursing
Manipal College of Nursing, Manipal, MAHE

Mrs Sweety Jousline Fernandes MSc (N)
Assistant Professor
Department of Obstetrics and Gynecological Nursing
Manipal College of Nursing, Manipal, MAHE

Contents

Content

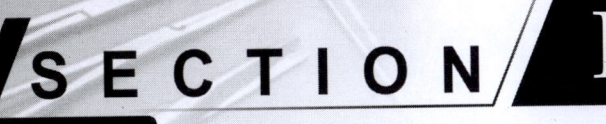

SECTION / I

Obstetric Drugs

1

Uterine Stimulants

Uterine stimulants are also referred to as uterotonics. These are medications given to initiate, increase the frequency and intensity of uterine contractions.

The common uterine stimulants used are:

1. Oxytocin
2. Prostaglandins
3. Ergot alkaloids

OXYTOCIN

Trade name: Pitocin, Syntocinon

Generic name: Oxytocin

Mechanism of action: Oxytocin, a hormone produced by the hypothalamus (paraventricular nuclei) is transported through nerve pathway to the posterior pituitary. It is released from the posterior pituitary by various stimuli from the cervix, the nipple, the vagina.

Oxytocin acts by modifying the cell membrane potential and inhibiting column binding in the sarcoplasmic reticulum, thereby increasing the intracellular free calcium and increasing its sensitivity. Oxytocin not only acts on the uterus but also acts on the breasts and kidneys.

Breasts: Oxytocin stimulates the myoepithelial cells and hence enables ejection of milk.

Kidneys: Due to its diuretic hormone like action, it causes a slight reduction of renal plasma flow due to constriction of afferent arterioles causing water intoxication.

Routes of administration: Intramuscularly/Intravenously

Dosage: Induction of labor

Intravenously: 0.5–1 milliunit/minute is used initially, gradually increase the dose in 30–60 minute intervals by increments of 1–2 milliunits/minute until desired contraction pattern is established (ACOG, 2009: Reaffirmed in 2016).

Uterine assessment prior to increasing the dose: In the previous 30 minutes all of the following conditions are met

- No more than 5 contractions in 10 minutes, averaged over the 30 minutes time period. No 2 contractions should be greater than 120 seconds in duration.
- The uterus palpates soft between contractions.
- If an intrauterine pressure catheter is in place (Montevideo units which is calculated by subtracting resting tone from peak uterine activity for each contraction in 10 minutes), must calculate less than 300 mm of Hg and the baseline intrauterine pressure resting tone must be less than 25 mm of Hg.

Fetal assessment prior to increasing the dose: In the previous 30 minutes all of the following conditions are met

- There is 1 acceleration of 15 bpm × 15 seconds, or there is moderate variability for 10 of the previous 30 minutes (FHR)
- No more than 1 late deceleration of FHR has occurred.
- No more than 2 variable deceleration of FHR exceeding 60 seconds in duration and decreasing greater than 60 bpm from the baseline have occurred.

Dosage: Postpartum bleeding:

- *Intramuscular:* Total dose of 10 units after delivery of the placenta.
- *Intravenous:* 10–40 units by IV infusion in 1000 ml of intravenous fluid at a rate sufficient to control uterine atony.

During abortion as adjunctive treatment

Intravenous: 10–20 milliunits/minute. Maximum total dose 30 units/12 hours.

Adverse reactions: Maternal

- *Cardiovascular:* Arrhythmias (including premature ventricular contractions), hypertensive episodes

Note: Factors to be assessed before administering oxytocin:
- The patientís pregnancy history and medical history
- Gestational age of the fetus
- Estimated fetal weight
- The fetal presenting part
- The adequacy of the pelvis
- The cervical status
- Clinical facilities are adequate to act in emergency

- *Gastrointestinal:* Nausea and vomiting
- *Genitourinary:* Pelvic hematoma, uterine hypertonicity, tetanic contraction of the uterus, uterine rupture, uterine spasm
- *Hematologic:* A fibrinogenemia (fatal)
- *Other reactions:* Anaphylactic reaction, subarachnoid hemorrhage, severe water intoxication with convulsions, coma and death is associated with a slow oxytocin infusion over 24 hrs.

Fetal/Neonatal
- *Cardiovascular:* Arrhythmias (including premature ventricular contractions), bradycardia
- *Central nervous system:* Brain or CNS damage, neonatal seizure.
- *Hepatic:* Neonatal jaundice
- *Ocular:* Neonatal retinal hemorrhage
- *Others:* Low Apgar score, fetal death.

Contraindications
- Hypersensitivity to oxytocin
- Significant cephalopelvic disproportion
- Malposition's and malpresentations
- Fetal distress
- Hypertonic or hyperactive uterus
- Vaginal deliveries in case of active genital herpes
- Invasive cervical cancer
- Cord presentation, prolapse of the cord
- Vasa previa or placenta previa
- Obstetrical emergencies where surgical interventions are needed.

Nurses responsibilities

1. Close monitoring of the mother and fetus for signs of hypertonic or hypotonic uterine contractions, water intoxication and hypersensitivity reaction.
2. Dosage to be carefully regulated to prevent adverse effects. Have magnesium sulfate (20% solution) available for relaxation of the myometrium in case there is hypertonic uterine contractions.
3. Intravenous preparations to be carefully administered by accurate calculation of dosage.
4. Monitor the uterine contractions. If uterine contractions are less than 2 minutes apart, if they were above 50 mm of Hg or if they last 90 seconds or longer then stop oxytocin infusion, turn the patient on her left side and notify the obstetrician.
5. Avoid use of oxytocin with carboprost tromethomine which may enhance the adverse/toxic effect of oxytocin.
6. Monitor urine output and vital signs specially BP, pulse and respiratory rate.

Administration protocol

- Oxytocin administration is initiated at a dose of 2 ml/U per minute.
- Without contraindication, the dose is increased by 2 m/U per minute every 30 minutes.

If above fetal criteria are not met: Reduce or stop oxytocin and perform patient assessment.

- Oxytocin is increased until there is normal progression of labor, or there are strong contractions occurring at 2–3 minute intervals.
- Oxytocin should be titrated to the lowest dose necessary for physiologic progress of labor. In some cases this will result in discontinuation after the onset of active labor.
- A numeric value for the maximum dose of oxytocin has not been established. Oxytocin may be increased until regular uterine contractions are established.

PROSTAGLANDINS

Prostaglandins (PG) are the derivatives of prostanoic acid, from which they get their names. They have a property of acting as 'local hormones'. Of many varieties of PGE_1, PGE_2, $PGF_{2\alpha}$ are exclusively used in obstetrics.

Uses of prostaglandins
- Induction of labor
- Termination of molar pregnancy
- Cervical ripening prior to induction of labor
- Management of atonic postpartum hemorrhage
- Management of tubal ectopic pregnancy.

Mechanism of action: PGE_2, $PGF_{2\alpha}$ have oxytocic effect on the gravid uterus, when used in appropriate doses they cause changes in myometrial cell membrane permeability and/or alteration of membrane bound calcium. PGE_2 is 5 times more potent than $PGF_{2\alpha}$.

Side effects
- Cervical lacerations
- Risk of uterine rupture
- Vomiting
- Pyrexia
- Tachycardia and chills
- Tachysytole
- Nausea
- Diarrhea
- Bronchospasm

PROSTAGLANDIN E_2

It is widely used because it is less toxic and more effective.

Trade name: Dinoprostone gel, Cerviprime gel, Primopost, Cervidil, etc.

Mechanism of action: Mainly acts on cervix causing ripening of cervix, making if softer and causing it to begin to dilate and efface. It also stimulates uterine contractions.

Dosage and route

Intravaginal 0.5 mg administered into cervical canal below the level of internal os of the cervix or 1–2 mg in the posterior fornix.

Vaginal tablets 3 mg administered into the posterior fornix followed by 3 mg after 6–8 hours.

Vaginal pessary (with retrieval device) releases dinoprostone approximately 10 mg over 24 hours. It is removed when cervical ripening is adequate.

Parenteral IV prostin E_2 containing 1 mg/ml.

If oral 0.5 mg is initially given, repeated hourly, should not exceed 1.5 mg.

Indications
- Cervical ripening
- Induction of labor
- To induce abortion

Side effects
- Headache
- Nausea
- Vomiting
- Fever
- Hypotension
- Fetal passage of meconium
- Amniotic fluid embolism during labor

Contraindications
- Hypersensitivity
- Patients in whom oxytocin is contraindicated
- Ruptured membranes
- Noncephalic presentation
- Previous caesarean section.

Nurses responsibilities
- Explain procedure of induction to the mother and her family in detail.
- Obtain informed consent
- Assess and document maternal and fetal well-being before and after administration by monitoring uterine contractions, fetal heart rate and vital signs.
- Use caution if the woman has history of asthma, glaucoma, renal, hepatic and cardiovascular disorders.

- Bring cerviprime gel to room temperature before administration.
- Assist woman to maintain supine position or side lying position and advice her to lie down for 30–60 minutes after administration of the gel.

PROSTAGLANDIN E$_1$

It is rapidly absorbed and more effective than oxytocin or dinoprostone for induction of labor.

1. Mifepristone (Mifeprex)
2. Misoprostol (Cytotec)

MIFEPRISTONE

Generic name: Mifepristone

Trade name: T-Pill, Mifegest, MFT, Mifebort syrup, Mt Pill, Abo Pill, Termipill, Mifeprin, Unwanted 72, Mefipil, etc.

Mechanism of action: Mifepristone is an antiprogestin which binds with progesterone receptor to block the receptor thereby inhibits progesterone from binding. It also softens and dilates the cervix, increases uterine lining prostaglandin release, enhances uterine contraction and causes decidual necrosis leading to placental detachment.

Indications

- Mifepristone is used for termination of pregnancy of less than 49 days.
- Used as an emergency contraceptive

Contraindications

- Chronic adrenal failure.
- Long term corticosteroid therapy
- Anticoagulant therapy or medications that interfere with hemostasis
- Hemorrhagic diseases.

Side effects

- Nausea
- Vomiting
- Abdominal pain
- Pelvic pain

Regimen: Common regimens—there are two protocols that are most common in practice

- US Food and Drug Association (FDA) approved/manufacturer recommended regimen—Mifepristone 600 mg orally, followed 48 hours later by misoprostol 400 µg orally.
- Alternative regimen—Mifepristone 200 mg orally followed by 24 to 72 hours and later by misoprostol 800 µg buccally.

MISOPROSTOL

It is one of the essential drug termed under World Health Organization because of its wide ranging application in reproductive health.

Generic name: Misoprostol

Trade name: Cytotec, Mifenac, Misonac, Safeguard

Mechanism of action: It is a synthetic prostaglandin E_1 (PGE_1) analog that causes cervical ripening.

Routes and dosage of administration: Oral, vaginal, sublingual, buccal and rectal.

Evidence based practice: Misoprostol for induction of labor at term
Recommendations (WHO guidelines)

1. Oral misoprostol (25 µg, 2-hourly) is recommended for induction of labor. (Moderate quality evidence, strong recommendation)
2. Vaginal low-dose misoprostol (25 µg, 6-hourly) is recommended for induction of labor. (Moderate quality evidence, weak recommendation)
3. Misoprostol is not recommended for women with previous caesarean section. (Low-quality evidence, strong recommendation)

Misoprostol for termination of pregnancy in women with a fetal anomaly or after intrauterine fetal death

For medical termination: 400 µg orally 48 hr after mifepristone administration.
800 µg vaginally 48 hr after mifepristone administration.

Labor induction or cervical ripening: 0.25 mg may repeat at intervals no more frequent than every 3–6 hours (ACOG, 2009)

Prevention of postpartum hemorrhage: Oral 600 µg as a single dose administered immediately after delivery, sublingual: 800 µg as a single dose (FIGO, 2012)

Indications

- To induce abortions
- Medical management of miscarriage
- To induce labor
- To prevent and treat postpartum hemorrhage
- Cervical ripening before procedures

Adverse effects: Diarrhea, abdominal pain, flatulence, nausea, headache, dyspepsia, vomiting and constipation.

Contraindications: The use of prostaglandins are not recommended in the following conditions/situations. (Wilson C, 2000)

- Noncephalic presentation
- Placenta previa
- Prolapsed umbilical cord
- Previous uterine surgery (of any kind)
- Chorioamnionitis
- Acute fetal distress
- Fever
- Bronchial asthma
- Epilepsy
- Hypersensitivity to drug, known patient allergy
- Renal disease
- Hypertension
- Peptic ulcer
- Estimated fetal weight > 4,500 g
- Labor (>12 contractions hr)
- Glaucoma, renal or hepatic disease

Nurses responsibilities

- Ensure that the informed consent is taken and the patient feelings are noted before induction.
- Assess and document the patient's vital signs (blood pressure, pulse, respirations) every 4th hourly to see if vital

signs are stable. Take a complete history in order to make sure that the patient meets the criteria (Bishop score of less than 6, cephalic presentation, and a reassuring fetal heart rate pattern 120–160 bpm) for labor induction. This will enable to ascertain the safety of misoprostol administration.

- Assess for inclusion factors to administer misoprostol. The other inclusion factors include maternal medical problems (e.g. diabetes) and a past date pregnancy.
- Assess for woman having contraindications. Misoprostol should not be administered to women with chorioamnionitis.
- The fetal factors that need to be evaluated to exclude misoprostol administration consist of multiple gestations, malpresentations, evidence of cephalopelvic disproportion, and estimated fetal weight of less than 1,800 grams. Other contraindications are transverse lie and prolapsed umbilical cord.
- The temperature should be obtained every 2 hours after rupture of membranes to monitor the patient for signs of chorioamnionitis.
- Monitor continuously the fetal movement and uterine activity for 2 hours following prostaglandin administration. The drug can be discontinued with a reassuring EFM tracing and in the absence of regular contractions (every 5 minutes).
- Liquid diet to be given to the woman during induction.

ERGOT ALKALOIDS

Ergot is a fungus that grows commonly on rye and less commonly on other grasses such as wheat. This fungus synthesizes many agents that include acetylcholine, histamine and also it stimulates alpha-adrenergic receptors, serotonin receptors. This chemical helps in reducing bleeding by causing constriction of the blood vessels.

METHERGINE
Drug name: Methylergometrine
Functional class: Oxytocics
Trade name: Methergine

Chemical class: Ergot alkaloid

Ergometrine is used in the third stage of labor for the management of postpartum hemorrhage. Before the administration, the fetus should be delivered and the possibility of twin gestation should be ruled out. Administration of drug may cause hyper stimulation of the uterus that may results in uterine tetany, decreased uteroplacental blood flow, uterine rupture, cervical and perineal lacerations, and amniotic fluid embolism.

Mechanism of action
- Stimulates contraction of uterine smooth muscles with an increase in frequency, tone and amplitude.
- It produces arterial vasoconstriction by stimulating the alpha receptors.
- It also causes constriction of vascular smooth muscles, decreases bleeding post-delivery.

Dosage and route
IM: 0.2 mg after the delivery as a prophylaxis against postpartum haemorrhage
IV: 0.2 mg given over/min

Indications
To shorten the duration of third stage of labor, routine management after the delivery of placenta to prevent postpartum postnatal atony and hemorrhage, uterine subinvolution, abortion or expulsion of hydatidiform mole, prophylaxis against excessive bleeding.

Adverse reaction: Confusion, coma, headache, dizziness, tinnitus, abdominal pain, nausea and vomiting, chest pain, hypertension, palpitation, hypotension, bradycardia, severe cramping, sweating, dyspnea, nasal congestion.

Contraindications
- Induction/augmentation of labor during delivery of live fetus (first and second stage)
- Hypertensive disorders of pregnancy (pre-eclampsia, eclampsia)
- Heart disease complicating pregnancy

- Peripheral vascular disease
- Rh negative pregnancy
- Hypersensitivity.

Nurses responsibilities

- Methergine should be administered alone because it may cause incompatibility with other drugs.
- Monitor and document vital signs, watch for changes in vitals that may indicate hemorrhage like falling BP, weak pulse.
- Assess fundal tone, check for relaxation of uterus or severe cramping.
- Assess for overdose, vomiting and nausea, muscular pain.
- Check calcium level before giving this drug.
- Restrict the administration through intravenous route in emergency because the risks of adverse effects are more. If intravenous route is used, it should be administered slowly or diluted with 5 ml sodium chloride and administered slowly over one minute.

Bibliography

1. Arias F, Daftary SN and Bhide AG (2008). Practical guide to high risk pregnancy and delivery (3rd ed.). Delhi: Elsevier.
2. Daftary SN. Chakravarthi, S (2011). Manual of Obstetrics (3rd ed.). New Delhi; Elsevier.
3. Dutta DC (2013). Textbook of Obstetrics (7th ed.). New Delhi: Jaypee.
4. Schiling J. Nursing Pharmacology. Philadelphia: Wolters Kluwer.
5. Weiner CP, Buhimschi C (2009). Drugs for pregnant and lactating Women (2nd ed.). Philadelphia: Saunders Elsevier.
6. Wilson C (2000). The Nurses' Role in Misoprostol Induction: A Proposed Protocol; Journal of Obstetric, Gynecologic and Neonatal Nursing, 29(6).
7. ACOG Committee on Practice Bulletins—Obstetrics, "ACOG Practice Bulletin No.107: Induction of Labor," Obstet Gynecol, 2009; 114 (2 Pt1): 386–97 [PubMed 19623003].
8. FIGO Guidelines: Prevention of PPH with misoprostol, 2012.

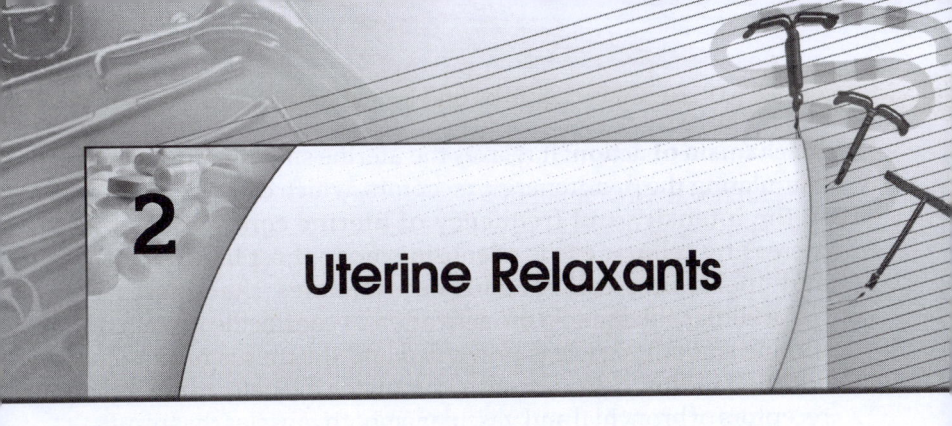

2

Uterine Relaxants

Tocolytic agents: Tocolytics are drugs to manage preterm labor which relaxes the smooth muscles of the uterus, thereby inhibits/suppresses uterine contractions, to safeguard against miscarriage after interventional obstetric procedures such as cervical encirclage, amniocentesis and cordocentesis.

Classification

1. Beta sympathomimetics (Ritodrine, isoxsuprine)
2. Calcium antagonists (Nifedipine)
3. Magnesium sulfate
4. Prostaglandin inhibitors (Indomethacin)

BETA SYMPATHOMIMETICS

Uterus has alpha receptors which mediate stimulant effects on the myometrium and beta receptors whose activation inhibits uterine contractions. Beta sympathomimetics act by stimulating beta receptors in the uterine muscles leading to reduction in the free intracellular calcium which is necessary for myometrial contraction.

RETRODRINE HYDROCHLORIDE

Drug name: Ritodrine hydrochloride

Trade name: Miolene, Ritodrine, Ritrod, Utgard

Functional class: It is a beta 2 adrenergic agonist

Pre-requisite: Tocolytic drugs should be used in spontaneous labor between 24 and 32 weeks of gestation, when the cervix is less than 4 cm dilated and membranes are intact.

Mechanism of action: It relaxes the uterine smooth muscles by stimulating the β_2-adrenergic receptors, which causes decrease in the intensity and frequency of uterine contractions by increasing cellular cyclic adenosine monophosphate (cAMP) and increasing cell membrane cytokines that increase intracellular calcium. So the activation of contractile protein of uterine smooth muscle is prevented and the uterus relaxes. In addition to this, Ritrodine also stimulates the beta-adrenergic receptors of bronchial and vascular smooth muscles that results in bronchodialation and increased heart rate.

Dosage and route

Intravenous: One ampoule contains 5 ml (50 mg), add 2 ampoules, i.e. 10 ml (10 mg/ml) in 500 ml of 5% dextrose solution and start infusion at a rate of 5 drops/minute for first 10 minutes and increase to 10 drops/minutes after that and continue for 10 more minutes. Drip rate is increased every 10–15 minutes by 5 drops/minute until uterine contractions stop. Once the uterine contractions ceases maintain drip rate for one hour, thereafter, continue the infusion for about 12 hours and later switch over to oral.

IM: 10 mg every 4–6 hr.

Oral: 120 mg daily 30–60 min before the termination of IV infusion with 10 mg every 2–6 hr.

Modified dose of drip: 5% dextrose, at a rate of 50–100 microgram/minute gradually increased until the contractions stop to a maximum.

Indication: Management of uncomplicated premature labor.

Side effects

Maternal:
- Shortness of breath
- Coughing
- Tachypnea
- Pulmonary edema
- Tachycardia
- Palpitation, chest pain
- Fluid retention

- Decreased urine output
- Tremors.

Fetal/neonatal
- Mild tachycardia
- Hyperglycemia
- Hyperbilirubinemia
- Hypertension

Contraindications
- Hypovolemia
- Bleeding
- Hypertension
- Thyroid dysfunction
- Cardiac disease of any kind
- Diabetes
- Chronic fetal distress
- Infections
- Antepartum hemorrhage
- Severe pregnancy induced hypertension, eclampsia, and pre-eclampsia
- Intrauterine fetal death

Nurses responsibilities
- Assess maternal electrocardiogram before the beginning of therapy
- Assess the mother for heart disease, uncontrolled diabetes mellitus, etc.
- Assess mother and fetal condition to obtain baseline information before beginning the therapy and before increasing the dose each time.
- Check vital signs every 2nd hourly.
- Discontinue infusion and notify a physician if mother exhibits tachycardia, chest pain, and dysthymia

DUVADILAN

Trade name: Duvadilan, Suprox, Suvadilan, Tidilan
Generic name: Isoxsuprine hydrochloride

Mechanism of action
- Acts directly on the vascular smooth muscles and causes peripheral vasodilation.
- Acts on the beta receptors which are present in the uterus and secrets the enzyme adenocyclase and reduces intracellular free calcium and inhibits activation of myosin light chain kinase (MLCK) which causes relaxation of the smooth muscles of the uterus.

Dose and Route
Oral: Available as 10 mg tablet. 20 mg to be taken orally 4–8th hourly until uterine activity ceases, thereafter, reduce the dose to 10 mg as clinically indicated.

Intramuscular: Starting with low dose of 5 mg and gradually increasing the subsequent doses up to 20 mg until the uterine contractions ceases.

Intravenous: Infused at a rate of 0.2 mg/minute.

Indications
- Inhibition of preterm labor
- Inhibition of uterine contraction for the relief of acute fetal distress from extreme uterine contraction during labor.

Contraindications
- Arterial hemorrhage
- Heart diseases
- Severe anemia
- Tachycardia
- Hypotension
- Premature separation of placenta

Side effects
- Nausea
- Vomiting
- Abdominal distress
- Tachycardia
- Hypotension

- Maternal pulmonary edema
- Allergic dermatitis
- Cardiac arrhythmias
- Acute respiratory distress syndrome
- Hyperglycemia
- Hypokalemia
- Lactic acidosis
- Maternal death (rarely)

Nurses responsibilities

- Check vitals and BP
- Assess and monitor the uterine contractions and fetal heart rate
- Observe for adverse effect of the drug
- Withhold the drug and notify the physician if any adverse effects are noted
- If dizziness occurs patient may require assistance with ambulating.

CALCIUM ANTAGONISTS

When calcium enters myometrial cells of uterus, the uterine muscle contracts and tightens. When calcium flows back out of the cell, the muscle relaxes. Calcium channel blockers work by preventing calcium from moving into the muscle cells of the uterus, making it not able to contract.

Generic name: Nifedipine

Trade name: Calbloc, Calnif Retard, Depicor, Nicardipine, Verapamil

Mechanism of action: It blocks calcium activated K^+ channels beta-adrenergic receptors which in turn inhibits premature uterine contraction. Antagonizes action of calcium within myometrial cells to reduce uterine contraction.

Side effects

- Headache
- Flushing
- Maternal tachycardia
- Nausea
- Fall in BP

Dosage:

Oral: 10–20 mg every 4–6 hr

1. High dose (gestation weeks between 24 and 34 weeks): 20 mg loading dose, daily 120–160 mg for 48 hours, followed by 80–120 mg daily up to 36 weeks.
2. Low dose: 10 mg loading dose, daily 60–80 mg for 48 hours followed by 60 mg daily up to 36 weeks.

Caution: Combined therapy with betamimetics or magnesium sulfate should be avoided.

Nurses responsibilities

- Monitor for maternal pulse and blood pressure every 30 minutes during first hour of administration and later every hourly for 2 hours.
- Continuous monitoring of uterine contractions.

MAGNESIUM SULFATE

Magnesium sulfate is the drug of choice for eclampsia. Magnesium blocks and decreases neuronal calcium influx and induces cerebral vasodilatation and dilates uterine artery. Magnesium acts to relax smooth muscle of uterus and results in vasorelaxation.

Trade name: Magnesium sulfate (Epsom salt)

Mechanism of action: It acts by inhibiting calcium ion at the motor end plate thus reducing calcium influx. Also decreases acetylcholine release and its sensitivity at neuromotor junction and decreases neuromuscular irritability including vasomotor and uterine irritability.

Indications

- Severe pre-eclampsia
- Eclmapsia
- Epilepsy

Side effects

- Flushing
- Perspiration

- Headache
- Muscle weakness
- Neonatal side effects include lethargy
- Hypotonia
- Respiratory distress

Contraindications

- Women with myasthenia gravis
- Heart block
- Myocardial damage
- Impaired renal function

Dosage

Intravenous bolus of 4–6 g (10–20% solution) over 20–30 minutes followed by an infusion of 1–2 g/hr. Continue at 1 g/hr for 4 hours and then cease $MgSO_4$ infusion.

Nurses responsibilities

Monitor the respiratory rate (one of the complication is respiratory muscle paralysis). If less than 10 breaths/min withhold the administration.

- Monitor maternal oxygen saturation every hourly
- Assess vital signs every 5–10 minutes
- Monitor serum magnesium level
- Monitor for overdosage
- Test knee-jerk reflex every 15 minutes for first 2 hours if found absent withhold the drug
- Monitor urine output hourly, if it drops below 25 ml/hr notify and do not repeat the next dose.

PROSTAGLANDIN INHIBITORS

Indomethacin: It is a cyclo-oxygenase inhibitor that prevents synthesis of prostaglandins. Indomethacin is given as a first line of treatment for women who have preterm contractions at 24–32 weeks of gestation.

Mechanism of action: Reduces synthesis of prostaglandins thereby reduces intracellular free calcium, activation of myosin light chain kinase (MLCK) which suppresses uterine contractions.

Dosage: Oral 50 mg followed by 25 mg every 6 hr for 48 hours for 2–3 days.

Side effects
- Heartburn
- Asthma
- GI bleeding
- Thrombocytopenia
- Renal impairment
- Platelet dysfunction

Contraindications
- Hepatic disease
- Active peptic ulcer
- Coagulation disorders

Nurses responsibilities
- Ensuring sonographic evaluation for oligohydramnios
- Ensuring sonographic evaluation for narrowing of fetal ductus arteriosis.

Tocolytics are administered to women with preterm labor at a gestational age at which a delay in delivery for 4–8 hours will provide benefit to newborn.

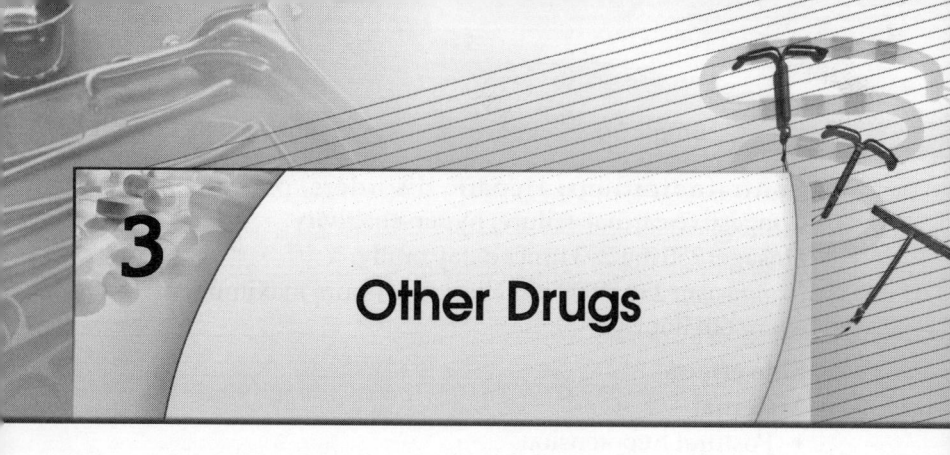

3

Other Drugs

ANTIHYPERTENSIVES

METHYLDOPA

Trade name: Alphadopa, Dopegyt, Emdopa, Aldomet

Chemical name: Centrally acting alpha adrenergic inhibitor

Functional class: α_2-adrenergic agonist and antihypertensive.

Mechanism of action: It stimulates alpha adrenergic receptors in the CNS resulting in decreased sympathetic outflow which decreases peripheral resistance and thereby helps in controlling blood pressure.

Pregnancy implications: Adverse reactions have not been reported in any of the studies conducted on animals. It is proved that it crosses the placenta and appears in cord blood. Evidences from the studies shows that use of methyldopa during pregnancy does not cause any harm to the fetus in turn it improves the fetal outcome. Methyldopa is a preferred drug for the treatment of chronic hypertension during pregnancy. In emergency situation if it is required to control the acute hypertension urgently, other forms of injectable antihypertensive agents are preferred.

Lactation: Excretes in breast milk. So it is advised to use this drug with caution. These infants should be monitored for adverse effects of the drug.

Indications: Pregnancy induced hypertension, hypertension, and hypertension crisis.

Contraindications: Hepatic disorders, psychic patients, Congestive cardiac failure, hypersensitivity.

Dosage: 250 mg 2–3 times a day orally.

IV infusion: 250–1000 mg every 6–8 hours maximum of 1gram every 6th hourly.

Side effects
Maternal
- Postural hypotension
- Hemolytic anemia
- Sodium retention
- Excessive sedation
- Constipation
- Weakness
- Giddiness
- Angina edema thrombocytopenia

Fetal: Intestinal ileus

Nurses responsibilities
1. Assess the blood values like complete blood count, mini liver function test, renal function test, etc. and electrocardiogram.
2. Monitor the blood pressure before the administration of medication each time.
3. Assess the urine output and monitor the intake output chart.
4. Advice the client not to discontinue or skip the drug abruptly without seeking medical advice.
5. Advice the client to get up slowly from the bed to prevent orthostatic hypotension.
6. Inform the client about the adverse reaction and side effects. Also inform about the sedative effect of the drug.
7. Monitor the complete blood count, liver function test and direct Coombs' test periodically.

AMLODIPINE
Trade name: Amlodipine

Functional class: Calcium channel blocker, antihypertensive

Chemical class: Dihydropyridine

Dose: 5 mg once daily, maximum dose up to 10 mg in a day.

Mechanism of action of the drug

It helps in inhibiting the calcium ion influx across cell membrane during cardiac depolarisation, also relaxes the coronary smooth muscles and peripheral vascular smooth muscles. It dilates the coronary arteries thereby increases the myocardial oxygen delivery.

Pregnancy implications: A few animal studies have shown adverse effects. Uncontrolled maternal hypertension results with fetal, neonatal and maternal mortality and morbidity. If treatment for hypertension in pregnancy is advised, other hypertensive drugs are preferred like Aldomet, labetalol, etc.

Lactation: Excretion of drug in breast milk is unknown, so it is usually not recommended during lactation.

Indications
- Chronic angina
- Hypertension
- Pregnancy induced hypertension (use cautiously)

Contraindications
- Hypersensitivity
- Severe aortic stenosis

Nurses responsibilities
1. Assess the vital signs, electrocardiogram before beginning the therapy.
2. Monitor intake output record, daily weight chart
3. Advice to take the drug as prescribed, not to double the dose or skip the dose.
4. To report immediately if any complications arise like shortness of breath, pedal edema and facial puffiness.
5. Assess the fetal heart rate frequently, monitor for daily fetal movement counts regularly.
6. Monitor the heart rate, blood pressure and peripheral edema. If a woman complains of having severe edema, consider switching over to other antihypertensive drug.

NIFEDIPINE

Trade name: Nifedipine

Chemical name: Calcium channel blocker, antihypertensive

Dose: 10–20 mg every 6th hourly

Mechanism of action: It prevents the calcium ions entry into the vascular smooth muscles and myocardium at the time of depolarisation, thereby causing relaxation of the coronary vascular smooth muscles and dilatation. This improves oxygen supply to the myocardium. Also, it helps in decreasing the peripheral vascular resistance and thus brings a reduction in blood pressure.

Pregnancy implications: Adverse effects were observed in many animal studies. Nifedipine crosses the placenta and increased incidence of perinatal asphyxia, cesarean delivery, and intra-uterine growth restriction have been noted following maternal use. Nifedipine is considered one of the best treatment option for treatment of hypertension during pregnancy (ACOG, 2013).

Lactation: Not recommended during lactation.

Indications: Hypertension, angina

Contraindications
- Hypersensitivity
- Acute myocardial infarction
- Cardiogenic shock

Side effects
- Flushing
- Dizziness
- Headache
- Nausea
- Heartburn
- Palpitation
- Hypotension
- Mood changes
- Fatigue
- Diarrhea
- Constipation

- Abdominal cramps
- Blurring of vision
- Dyspnea

Midwives responsibilities

1. Assess the vital signs and monitor the blood pressure every 2nd hourly and before the administration of each dose.
2. Monitor intake output chart
3. Advice to take the drug as prescribed, not to double the dose or skip the dose.
4. To report immediately if any complications like heartburn, palpitation blurring of vision dyspnoea arise and to notify the physician.
5. Assess the fetal heart rate frequently, monitor for daily fetal movement counts regularly.
6. Monitor every 4th hourly heart rate, signs and symptoms of congestive heart failure and peripheral edema.

LABETALOL

Trade name: Labetalol

Functional class: Antihypertensive

Chemical class: Beta blocker with alpha-blocking activity

Dose: Oral: Initially 100 mg twice daily, can be increased as needed every 2 to 3 days by 100 mg twice daily (titration should not exceed 200 mg in total) until desired response is obtained.

IV bolus: Initially 20 mg IV over 2 minutes; repeat 40 to 80 mg at 10-minute intervals, maximum up to 300 mg. After the initial loading dose infusion can be started at a rate of 1–2 mg/minute.

Mechanism of action of the drug: Labetalol blocks the adrenergic receptors thus helps in expanding the arteries which results in fall in the blood pressure.

Pregnancy implications: Adverse effects with the use of labetalol have been reported from the animal reproduction studies. Labetalol cross the placenta and it can be noted in the cord blood and serum of the infants after delivery. Use of labetalol during pregnancy increases the risk of fetal/neonatal bradycardia; hypoglycaemia, hypotension and respiratory depression. Oral administration of labetalol is considered best for the treatment of chronic hypertension of pregnancy and intravenous administration is advised for pre-eclampsia and eclampsia and postpartum eclampsia where immediate control of blood pressure is expected. It is advised to avoid the use of labetalol in women with asthma or heart failure.

Lactation: Low amounts of labetalol are found to be excreted in breast milk and hence it is advised to use with caution in lactating mothers.

Indications
- Chronic hypertension
- Pre-eclampsia
- Eclampsia
- Pregnancy induced hypertension
- Postpartum hypertension.

Contraindications
- Hypersensitivity
- Asthma
- Heart diseases

Side effects
- Dizziness
- Tingling scalp or skin
- Light headedness
- Excessive tiredness
- Headache
- Stomach upset
- Stuffy nose
- Chest pain
- Edema
- Shortness of breath
- Wheezing

Nurses responsibilities
1. Assess the vital signs and monitor the blood pressure regularly before the administration of medication each time.

2. Investigations like complete blood count, liver and renal function test, electrocardiogram should be done prior to beginning of the medication and should repeat biweekly.
3. Monitor intake output chart
4. Advice to take the drug as prescribed, not to double or skip the dose.
5. To report immediately if any complications arise and to notify the physician of symptoms like edema wheezing chest pain, sudden weight gain, shortness of breath.
6. Assess the fetal heart rate frequently, monitor for daily fetal movement counts regularly.
7. Monitor regularly the heart rate, signs and symptoms of congestive heart failure and peripheral edema and weight chart.

HYPOGLYCEMIC AGENTS

Diabetes mellitus (DM) is characterised by hyperglycaemia due to absolute or relative deficiency of insulin. Deficiency of insulin interferes with the metabolism of carbohydrates, fat and protein.

INSULIN

Trade name: Insulin regular, Insulin lispro, Insulin aspart

Chemical name: Humulin R, Novolin R

Mechanism of action: Insulin is a naturally produced hormone in our body which is secreted by the pancreas. It helps in decreasing blood glucose by transporting glucose into cells thus converting the glucose into glycogen; also indirectly it helps in increasing pyruvate and lactate and decreasing the phosphate and potassium.

Pregnancy Implications

Insulin is considered as the drug of choice for treating diabetes during pregnancy. Insulin therapy should be considered in pregnant women if the women fail to maintain the glucose levels after the initiation of diet therapy. Dosage and timing of administration should be adjusted by frequently monitoring the blood glucose levels. Minimal amount of endogenous insulin croses the placenta. Insulin requirement is less during the first trimester and the requirement is increased in second and third trimester especially between 28 to 32 weeks of gestation. Following delivery insulin requirement decreases rapidly because of lower insulin resistance. Poorly controlled diabetes may affect the pregnancy outcome.

Lactation: During lactation insulin levels drops because of increased metabolic demand. Excretion of insulin in breast milk is unknown.

Indications: Type I and Type II diabetes mellitus, gestational diabetes mellitus, diabetic ketoacidosis.

Contraindication: Hypersensitivity

Side effects

Hypoglycaemia: It is the most common and fatal complication and can occur in any diabetic client. It may be due to delay in taking food after the insulin administration, heavy physical activity and high dose of insulin.

A person with hypoglycemia may exhibit following symptoms: Confusion, anxiety, tremor, tachycardia, tiredness, perspiration, headache, palpitation, blurred vision, loss of consciousness, convulsions.

Other side effects are
- Lipodystrophy
- Lipohypertrophy
- Edema due to salt and water retention

Nurses responsibilities

1. Advice the client to note the fetal movements for about an hour after breakfast, lunch and dinner and to report immediately if the total counts are less than ten.
2. Advice to keep the insulin kit available at all times
3. Always carry candy or sugar to treat hypoglycemia and to carry diabetic ID. It may help in identifying the symptoms and complications at the earliest.
4. Advice regarding the symptoms of hypo and hyperglycemia and ketoacidosis, it will help the client to identify the manifestations at the earliest.

5. The dosage, route and site of administration, dietary restrictions need to be clearly instructed to the clients at the beginning of the therapy.
6. Advice regarding follow-up: About glucose testing to determine the effectiveness of treatment.

METFORMIN

Trade name: Metformin

Functional category: Oral antidiabetic

Chemical name: Biguanide

Mechanism of action: It inhibits the hepatic glucose production and increases the peripheral tissue sensitivity to insulin.

Pregnancy Implications

Adverse events have not been reported in any of the studies conducted on animals. It has been found to cross the placenta which may be comparable to those found in the maternal plasma. Also it is suggested to adjust the dosage of drug when it is recommended in third trimester. The studies are still going on to weigh the benefits of using metformin in pregnant women with Type II diabetes or GDM.

Lactation: Metformin excretes in breast milk, hence it is not recommended.

Indications: Type 2 DM, GDM

Contraindications
- Hypersensitivity
- Liver diseases
- Alcoholism
- Cardiopulmonary disease
- Myocardial infarction
- Diabetic ketoacidosis
- Metabolic acidosis

Side effects
- Headache
- Weakness

- Dizziness
- Drowsiness
- Tinnitus
- Fatigue
- Vertigo
- Heart failure
- Hypoglycemia
- Nausea
- Vomiting
- Diarrhea
- Anorexia
- Thrombocytopenia
- Rash

Nurses responsibilities

1. Assess for hypo-/hyperglycaemic reactions.
2. Check periodically blood sugar levels including liver function test, and complete blood count.
3. Advice to take the drug as prescribed preferably before meals.
4. Advice the client to note the fetal movements regularly and to report immediately if the counts are less than ten in a day.
5. Always carry candy or sugar to treat hypoglycaemia and to carry diabetic ID. It may help in identifying the symptoms and complications at the earliest.

MISCELLANEOUS

BETAMETHASONE/DEXAMETHASONE

Drug name: Betamethasone/Dexamethasone

Trade name: Betamethasone, sodium sulfate, bethosol, clistone, cortisol.

Chemical class: Long acting glucocorticoid

Action: It is used in pregnant woman to stimulate maturity of fetal lung by promoting release of enzymes that enhance production of lung surfactant in preterm labor.

Dosage and route
- 12 mg IM 12 hours apart two doses (dexamethasone).
- Betamethasone: 12 mg IM 24 hours apart two doses.

Indications
Prevent or reduce the severity of respiratory distress syndrome in preterm infants between 24 to 34 weeks of gestation.

Side effects
- There are no sources in the current document.
- Possible maternal infection—pulmonary edema, if given with beta adrenergic medications. It may worsen maternal condition like diabetics and hypertension.

Contraindication: It is contraindicated in women who are taking phenytoin or indomethacin.

Nurses responsibilities
- Give deep IM in gluteal muscles.
- Assess blood glucose level and lung sounds in between and after the administration of the drug.
- Do not give if the woman has infections
- Asses the mother for mood changes, behavioral changes, aggression.
- Assess for uterine tone and fetal heart rate.

VITAMIN K

Drug name: Vitamin K

Functional class: Vitamin K, fat-soluble vitamin

Trade name: Menadione sodium bisulfate, phytomenadione phosphate

Mechanism of action: For adequate blood clotting factors (II, VII, IX, X). The intestinal flora of newborn is sterile and starts producing vitamin K during first week of life, hence vitamin K is administered to promote formation of clotting factors in the liver.

Dosage and route
IM 1 mg (0.1 ml) given within 2 hours of birth.

Indication
Prevention and treatment of hemorrhagic disease in newborn.

Adverse reactions

- Edema
- Erythema
- Pain at injection site
- Hemolysis
- Jaundice
- Hyperbilirubinemia
- Sweating
- Flushing

Nurses responsibilities

1. Administer into mid anterior thigh, i.e. vastus lateralis muscle using tuberculine syringe and 25 gauge needle.
2. Observe for signs of oozing, petechiae, bleeding.

Bibliography

1. ACOG (2013). Hypertension in pregnancy. Report of the American College of Obstetricians and Gynecologists' Task Force on Hypertension in Pregnancy. Obstet Gynecol;122(5): 1122–1131.

2. http://www.uptodate.com/contents/ergonovine-drug information? source=search_result&search=ergometrine&selectedTitle=1~40.

3. Kalra P, Analkal M (2013). Peripartum management of diabetes. Indian Journal of Endocrinol Metab;17(7): 72–76.

4. Qarmalawi et al (1995). Labetalol vs. methyldopa in the treatment of pregnancy-induced hypertension. International Journal of Gynecology and Obstetrics; 49(2):125–130.

5. Roth LS (2015). Mosby's "Nursing Guide for Drug Reference" (10th ed.). Elsevier.

6. Tiziani A (2013). Havard's Nursing Guide to Drugs, Mosby Publication. Australia.

7. White WB et al (1985). "Alpha-Methyldopa Disposition in Mothers with Hypertension and in Their Breast-fed Infants." Clin Pharmacol Ther;37(4):387–390.

8. www.Cochranelibrary.com:http://onlinelibrary.wiley.com/o/ cochrane/clcentral/articles/099/CN-01007099/frame.html.

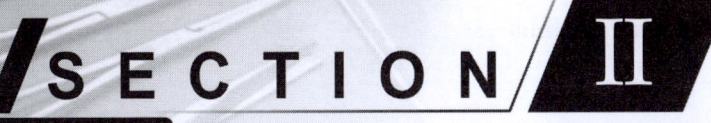

SECTION II

Contraception

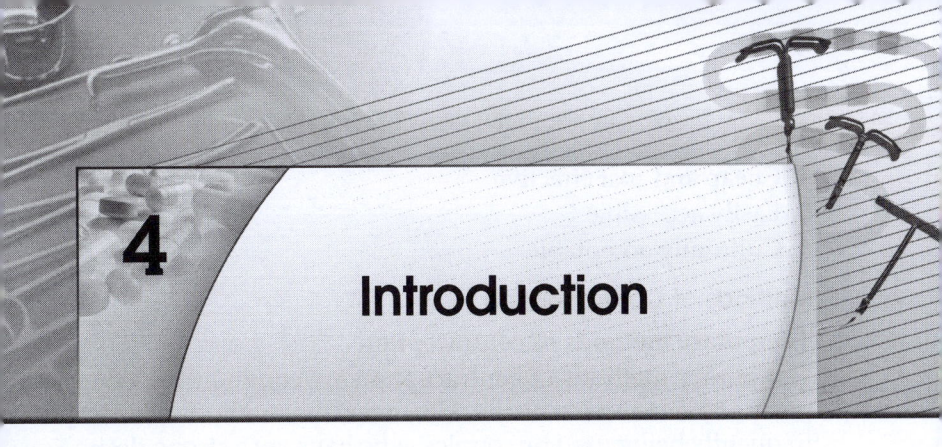

4

Introduction

Contraceptive methods, by definition, are preventive methods to help women avoid unwanted pregnancies. A method which is suitable for one group may not be suitable for another group because of one's different cultural patterns, religious beliefs and socioeconomic environment. The present approach is like a "cafeteria choice" where the couples are provided with the list of contraceptives and they have to select the best suitable for them, in view of preventing pregnancy.

Contraception and fertility control are not synonymous. Fertility control includes both fertility inhibition and fertility stimulation. While the fertility stimulation is related to the problem of the infertile couples, it includes temporary and permanent method intended to prevent pregnancy. Contraception means preventing the union of sperm and ovum, i.e. suppressing ovulation and interfering with implantation of the fertilized ovum in the uterus.

Best contraceptive methods must fulfil some criteria:
- It should be safe
- Simple to use
- Inexpensive
- Widely acceptable
- Highly effective
- Less motivation and supervision

Merits of good quality contraceptives
1. It should be 100 percent effective.
2. Free from side effects and complications
3. Return to fertility when discontinued

4. Cheap and cost effective
5. Easily accessible
6. Culturally acceptable

Methods of Contraception

Temporary methods of contraception

Temporary methods of contraception are commonly used to postpone or to space births. However, the methods are also frequently being used by couples, who have got a strong desire for no more children.

The temporary methods of contraception include:

1. Natural methods
2. Barrier methods
3. Intrauterine contraceptive devices (IUDs)
4. Hormonal methods

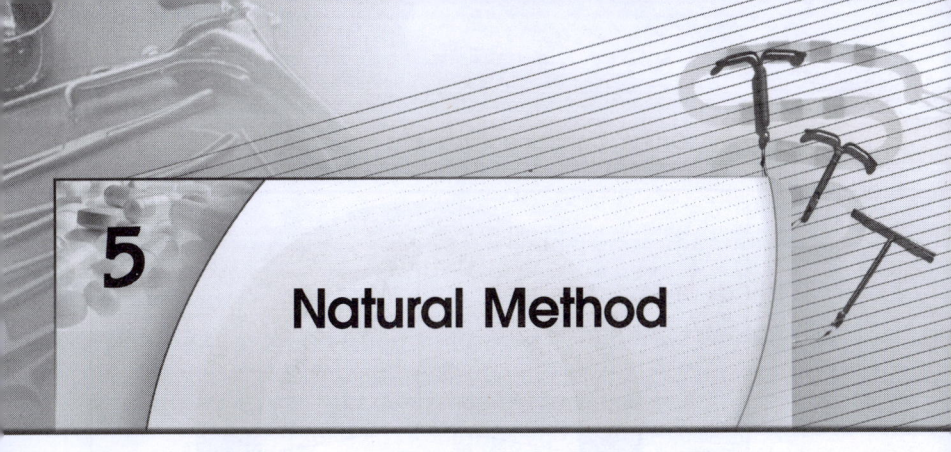

5

Natural Method

Natural family planning is also called periodic abstinence methods; it involves no introduction of foreign or chemical material into the body or abstaining from sexual intercourse during a fertile period. Fertility awareness methods are not costly but it require partner's cooperation. Also, the woman should know the fertile time of her menstrual cycle.

Natural methods are
- Abstinence during the fertile period
- Calendar/Rhythm method
- Cervical mucous method
- Basal body temperature method
- Symptothermal method
- Breastfeeding (lactation amenorrhea method)
- Withdrawal (coitus interruptus)

Abstinence during the fertile phase
It means fertility awareness the woman knows when the fertile period starts and when it ends. The fertile period of the menstrual cycle can be predicted by various methods.

Calendar/Rhythm Method
This is the only method approved by the Roman Catholic Church. The method is based on Knaus-Ogino theory which states ovulation occurs on day 14 ± 2 in a female with a regular 28 days cycle (so the couple has to avoid sex between 12th to the 16th day). But fertilizable span of sperm is 48–72 hours and ovum is 12–24 hours. Therefore, unsafe period is 8–19 days.

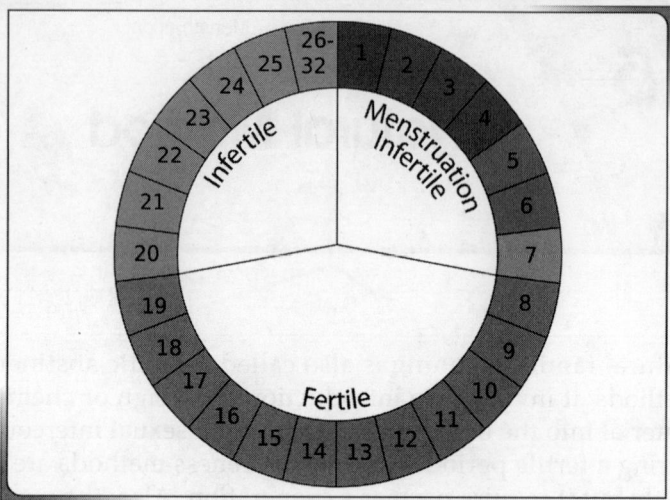

Fig. 5.1: Rhythm method

Therefore, safe period is calculated from the first day of the menstrual period until the 10th day of the cycle and from the 18th to the 28th day of cycle.

Failure rate can be reduced if sex is avoided from 7 to 21 days (failure rate 10%). Thus sex is safe only in the first and last 7 days of menstrual cycle.

In irregular cycle
- Subtract 18 from the shortest menstrual cycle (28–18 = 10)
- Subtract 11 from the longest menstrual cycle (32–11 = 21)
- Days 10–21 fertile period so couple should abstain from intercourse.

Advantage: Low cost and lack of side effects

The drawbacks of this method
1. If the cycles are irregular, it is difficult to predict the safe period.
2. "Planned sex" may be difficult for the couple.
3. This method is not applicable during the postnatal period.
4. High failure rate are due to wrong calculation and irregular menstrual cycles.

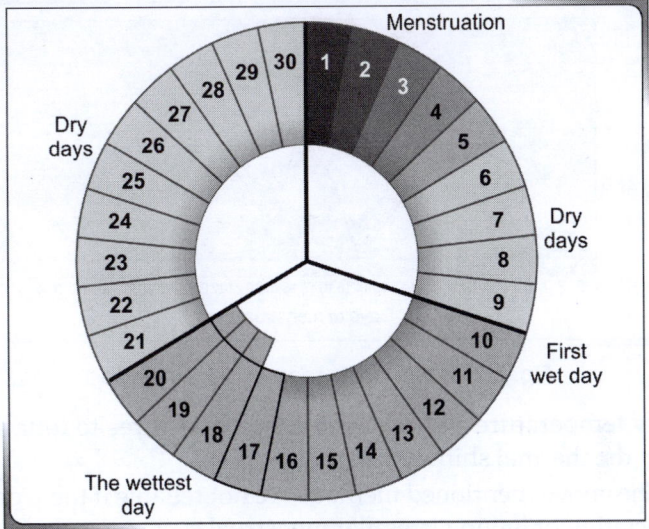

Fig. 5.2: Cervical Mucus method

Methods to determine the approximate time of ovulation and the fertile period include

Cervical mucus method: The cervical mucus changes based on the hormonal changes (i.e. ovarian and oestrogen) on the different days of the menstrual cycle. The women predict the fertile period by feeling the cervical mucus. The mucus is copious, slippery and increases in quantity till the peak period, and then it becomes thicker, dry and scanty till the onset of menstruation, under the influence of the hormone progesterone.

Basal body temperature method

The woman records her basal body temperature daily in the morning and then records it in the basal body temperature chart. If the temperature rises the woman should understand it is the time of ovulation due to the hormone progesterone. So, she should avoid intercourse during that period and thus prevent pregnancy.

Symptothermal method (Basal body temperature + cervical secretion)

This method is a combination of both the calendar and mucus method, whichever comes first. The woman checks her basal

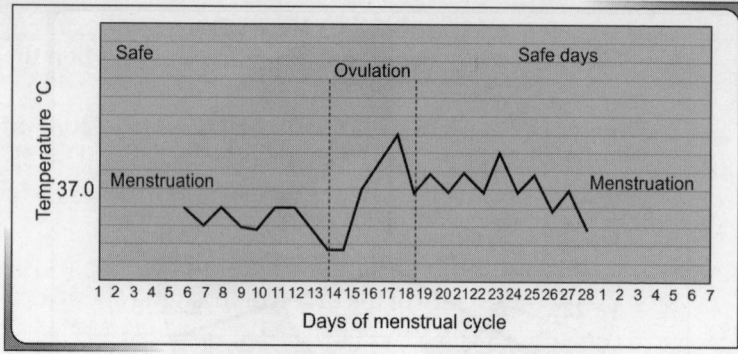

Fig. 5.3: Basal body temperature method

body temperature and resumes intercourse three to four days after the thermal shift.

The above mentioned methods are not reliable if the woman is lactating or having irregular menstrual cycles.

Breastfeeding (lactation amenorrhea method)

Prolonged and sustained breastfeeding offers a natural protection from pregnancy. It is more effective in women who have amenorrhea than those who are menstruating. The pregnancy rate for women who is fully breastfeeding and having amenorrhea is 2% in the first 6 months of exclusive breastfeeding. Otherwise failure rate is 1–10%, so additional contraceptive support should be given to the woman.

Withdrawal method/Coitus interruptus

It is the oldest and common practice, the coitus takes place normally but the penis is withdrawn immediately before ejaculation. Then the man withdraws and sperms are emitted outside the vagina.

Effectiveness: It is only about 75% effective because if sperms are present in the pre-ejaculation fluid, the fertilization may occur. (Stubblefield, Carr-Ellis, & Kapp, 2007).

Advantages

1. No contraindications and side effects
2. No effect on lactation
3. Failure rate—20–30%

Disadvantages

1. Requires sufficient self-control by the man
2. Not applicable during lactational amenorrhoea or when the periods are irregular
3. Failure rate of 19%, since pre-ejaculatory fluid may contain sperm.
4. The woman may develop anxiety neurosis, vaginismus or pelvic congestion.
5. Higher rate of ectopic or congenital abnormality of the foetus. Because of chance of the union of the aging sperm and ovum.
6. High failure rate and require more motivation
7. No protection against sexually transmitted diseases (STD) and human immunodeficiency virus (HIV) infection.

Effectiveness: The effectiveness of these methods varies greatly from 25 to 85%, depending mainly on the couple's ability to refrain from having sexual relations during the fertile period.

6

Barrier Method

Barrier methods do not allow the sperm to get deposited in the vagina, so prevent mobility of the sperm into the cervical canal.

Barrier methods are suitable for both men and women. It has dual role in prevention of pregnancy and STDs. The methods include placement of a chemical or other barrier between the cervix and the advancing sperms so that the sperms cannot enter the uterus or fallopian tubes and fertilize the ovum.

Mechanical Barriers

1. Male condom
2. Female condom, diaphragm, cervical cap.
3. Chemical (vaginal contraceptive)—Creams—Delfen
4. Foam tablets
5. Sponge (today)

Condom (Male)

Male condoms are a thin, flexible sheath or cover that is placed over the penis to prevent semen from entering the partner's body during sexual intercourse. Condoms can be either polyurethane or latex. Polyurethane condoms are thinner (0.010–0.020 mm) and suitable to those who are sensitive to latex rubber.

To help ensure optimal effectiveness and protection, people who use condoms must carefully follow instructions for their use. Before using a condom make sure it is not past its expiry date.

Spermicidal condoms (those that are packaged with spermicide applied to the condom) are not more effective and they expire faster than condoms without spermicide, and therefore are not recommended.

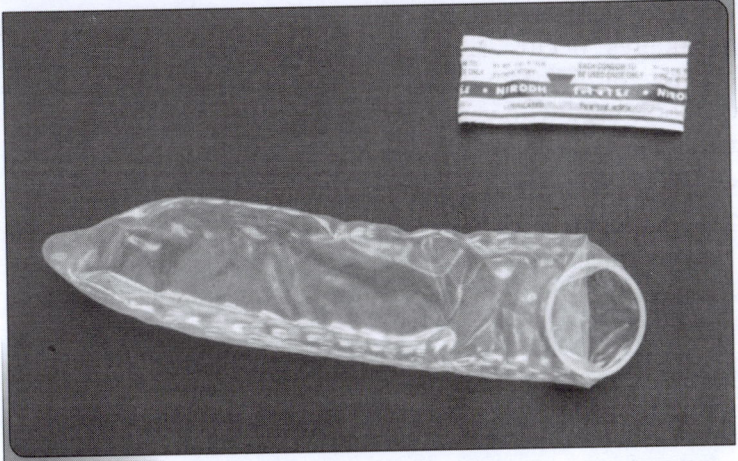

Fig. 6.1: Male condom

Advantages
1. Cheap and easily available
2. Safe and inexpensive
3. Easy to use; do not require medical supervision
4. Free from side effects
5. It has a duel role as a contraceptive and prevents STDs
6. It also prevents spread of dreaded HIV infections

Disadvantages
1. Partially reliable, having pregnancy rate of 10 to 15 per 100 women due to low quality
2. Lack of satisfaction
3. May cause allergy, as some people are allergic to latex
4. Some quality condom's used to prevent vaginal irritation are very expensive

Evidence based Practice
Condom effectiveness depends on the skill level and experience of the user. The use of a male condom and a full dose of vaginal spermicide (not a spermicide coated condom) theoretically reduces the overall risk of contraceptive failure, assuming that the contraceptive mechanisms of condoms and spermicides operate independently. A synergistic effect from lubricant

effects of spermicides may also be possible if fewer condom breakages occur. However, no trials have compared contraceptive effectiveness of condoms used alone versus condoms used with vaginal spermicide (Warner L, Steiner MJ male condoms, 2011).

Strategies for promoting effective condom use

1. **Effective use of condoms depends on the skill level and experience of the user.**
2. **Emphasize that condoms should be used with every coital act.**
3. **Instruct the client on use:** Encourage inexperienced clients to practice using condoms on a model of a penis.
4. **Inform the client to use the condom during the entire sexual act.**
5. **Discuss what to do if a condom slips or breaks:** Emergency contraception, now available over the counter without a prescription, can be used as a back-up method against pregnancy in case a condom breaks or falls off.
6. **Discuss use of lubricants and medications:** Clients should be aware of whether products they use (lubricants, medications) condoms contain oil. Spermicides are water-based. Other vaginal medications, however, often contain oil-based ingredients that can damage latex condoms.

Use of condoms

- An elective contraceptive method
- As an interim form of contraception during pill use, following vasectomy operation and if an IUD is thought to be lost until a new IUD can be fitted.
- During the treatment of trichomonal vaginitis of the wife, the husband should use it during the course of treatment.
- Immunological infertility—male partner to use for three months.

Advantages

- Cheap and no side effects
- Simple to use and easily disposable.
- Protection against STD and pelvic inflammatory diseases (PIDs).

- Protection against incidence of ectopic pregnancy and cervical cancer
- Useful where the coital act is infrequent and irregular.

Disadvantages
- May accidently break or slip of during coitus.
- Less sexual pleasure
- Failure rate is high if not used correctly.

Precautions
- Not to be used after the expiry date
- To cover the penis with condom prior to genital contact.
- To grasp the open end of the condom and hold it in place during withdrawal.

Side Effect and Contraindication
There are no contraindications to the use of condoms except for sensitivity to latex.

Female Condom

Female condoms are also known as a Femidom device made-up of a latex pouch with polyurethane and spermicide. The inner ring covers the cervix, and the external ring remains outside the vagina. It may be inserted at any time before the sexual activity

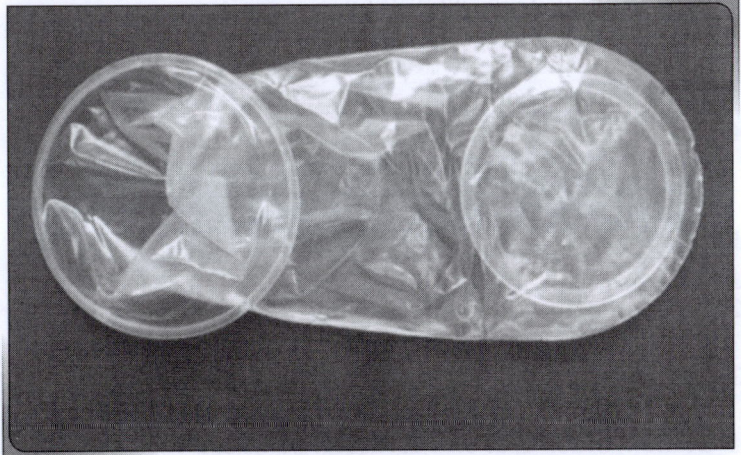

Fig. 6.2: Female condom

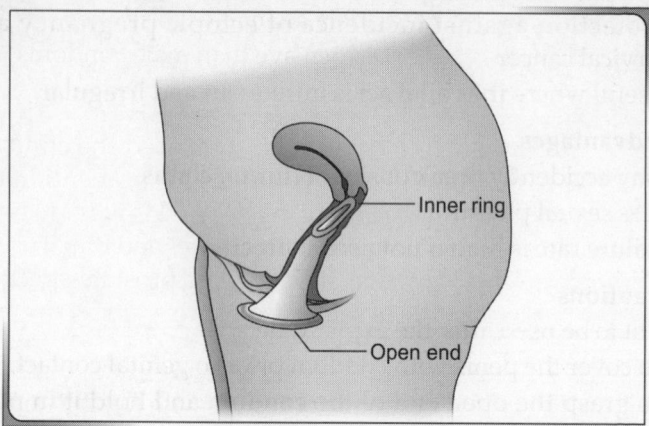

Fig. 6.3: Female condom, the inner ring keeps the condom in place

and removed after sexual activity. Like male condoms, it is used for one time and it offers dual protection against contraception and STDs.

Advantages
1. It is a safe, effective, reversible method of contraception with no delay in return of fertility following discontinuation of the method.
2. It can be obtained without a medical examination, prescription, or special fitting.
3. Its use is associated with minimal side effects since it is relatively inert and the body is exposed to it only in anticipation of coitus, not at other times.
4. It provides protection against STIs and offers an option to at-risk women whose partners cannot or will not use the male condom.

Disadvantages
1. Some women find it difficult to insert and remove.
2. The outer ring is visible outside the vagina, which can be unacceptable to either partner.
3. It has a higher failure rate in preventing pregnancy than nonbarrier methods and the male condom.
4. Some women feel embarrassed or uncomfortable when obtaining condoms or suggesting use of condoms.

5. Female condoms are not widely available worldwide.

6. Female condoms are more expensive than male condoms

Effectiveness

No published randomized trials have compared the clinical effectiveness of male and female condoms for prevention of either pregnancy or STIs (including HIV). However, two randomized crossover trials in the United States and Brazil used the proxy measures of breakage, slippage, and prostate-specific antigen (PSA) as indicators of semen exposure.

Diaphragm

It is an intra-vaginal device made of rubber with flexible metal or spring ring at the margin, its diameter varies from 5 to 10 cm. It has a flexible rim made of spring or metal. It is important that a woman be fitted with a diaphragm of the proper size. The distance between the tip of the middle finger placed in the posterior fornix and the point over the finger below the symphysis pubis gives approximate diameter of the diaphragm. Diaphragm should completely cover the cervix. As it cannot effectively prevent ascent of the sperms alongside the margin of the device, additional chemical spermicidal agent should be placed on the superior surface of the device during insertion, so that it remains in contact with the cervix. The device is introduced 3 hours before a sexual activity, and is kept in place

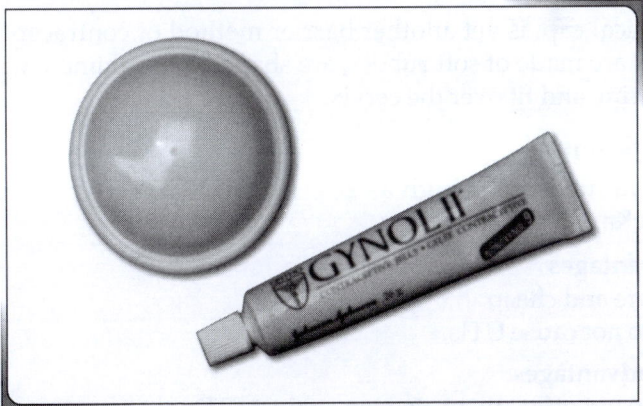

Fig. 6.4: Diaphragm with a spermicidal agent

for 6 hours. Ill-fitting and accidental displacement during intercourse increases the failure rate. Overall failure rate is 6–16%.

Advantages
- Cheap
- Can be used repeatedly for a long time.
- Used with spermicide reduces the incidence of PIDs/ STDs to some extent.

Disadvantages
- Requires help of a doctor or paramedical person to measure the size required
- Risk of vaginal irritation and UTIs
- Not suitable for women with uterine prolapse

Side effects and contraindication

Diaphragms may not be effective if the uterus is prolapsed, retroflexed or anti-flexed. Intrusion on the vagina by a cystocele or rectocele makes insertion of a diaphragm difficult.

Contraindications
- Toxic shock syndrome.
- Allergy to Latex and spermicides
- Recurrent urinary tract infections.
- Difficulty or discomfort with the insertion process
- High-risk of acquiring sexually transmitted infections

Cervical Cap

Cervical cap, is yet another barrier method of contraception. Caps are made of soft rubber, are shaped like a thimble with a thin rim, and fit over the cervix.

Effectiveness

The failure rate is high as 26% (ideal) to 32% (typical use) (MacKay, 2009).

Advantages
- Safe and cheap
- Do not cause UTIs.

Disadvantages
- Do not offer any protection against STDs.
- Difficult to insert the cap

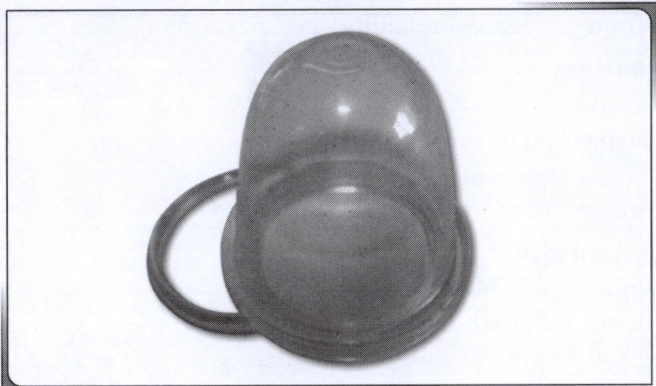

Fig. 6.5: Cervical cap

- Failure rate is more if not inserted correctly.
- It contains spermicides, which may lead to allergic reactions.

Contraindications
- Short and long cervix
- Abnormal pap smear
- History of toxic shock syndrome
- Any allergic reaction may lead to vaginal bleeding, cervicitis.
- Human papilloma viral (HPV) infection
- History of cervical cancer

Effectiveness
Cervical cap is less effective than other barrier methods. It has effective only, it used along with spermicide because the barrier function between the cap and the cervix is less secure than with a diaphragm. In a systematic review that included one trial of nearly 800 women, the six-month typical-use pregnancy rates were higher for Fem Cap users than for diaphragm users (Gallo MF, Grimes DA, Cochrane Database Systematic Rev. 2002).

Chemical Barriers (Vaginal Contraceptives)
A spermicide (Nonoxynol-9 or octoxynol-9 or Benzalkonium chloride), spermicides are available in many types; like, tablet, foam, jelly, cream and suppository. It is an agent that causes sperm immobilization and death of spermatozoa before they

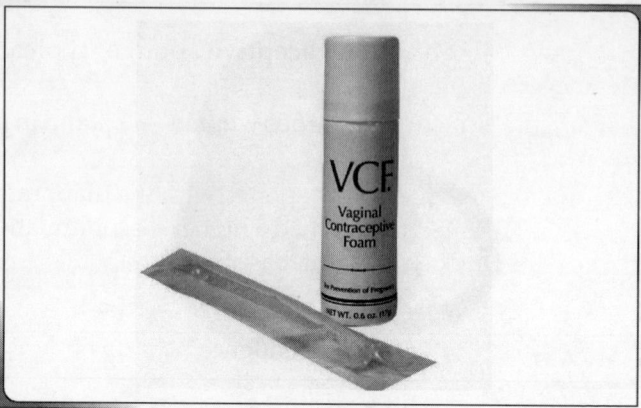

Fig. 6.6: Vaginal contraceptive foam tablets

can enter the cervix. Spermicidal changes the vaginal pH to a strong acid level, which is not conductive to sperm survival. However, they do not protect against STIs. The cream or jelly is introduced high in the vagina with the help of an applicator soon before coitus. Foam tablets (1or 2) are to be introduced high in the vagina at least 5 minutes prior to the sexual intercourse. In isolation, it is not effective but enhances the efficacy of condom or diaphragm when used along with it. There may be occasional local allergic manifestations either in the vagina or vulva.

Vaginal contraceptive sponge (Today)

The contraceptive sponge, commercially available as the Today Sponge, is a 2-inch wide foam disk, three-quarters of an inch thick, that contains 1000 mg of nonoxynol-9 and has a nylon loop attached to the bottom for removal. The sponge also contains sulfa and polyurethane. As of 2016, the Today Sponge is the main contraceptive sponge in production and is available in only one size and material. Because the sponge is sold over-the-counter and does not require a pelvic exam, it is a readily available option for women who desire immediate female-controlled contraception. The sponge releases spermicide during coitus, absorbs ejaculate and blocks the sperms' entrance to the cervical canal. The sponge should not be removed for 6 hours after intercourse.

Efficacy

For women using the contraceptive sponge, typical—use pregnancy rates are:

Failure rate is about nulliparous women—12% and in parous women—24%.

In a trial that compared the sponge with the diaphragm, the sponge was less effective and had a higher discontinuation rate (Kuyoh, M, 2002 Cochrane Database Syst Rev).

Advantages

- They allow for greater independence
- Lower cost
- Available in variety of brands

Disadvantages

- Effectiveness is least if not combined with barrier methods
- Failure rate is more
- Allergy to spermicide
- Increased risk of UTIs
- If frequently used this may cause genital lesions and increases risk of transmission of HIV.

Side Effects and Contraindications

1. Allergy or sensitivity to the chemicals in the product, particularly nonoxynol-9.
2. Vaginal and penile irritation is not uncommon with spermicide use
3. Spermicides do not protect against sexually transmitted infections
4. Spermicide-induced local mucosal inflammation, which reduces mucosal immunity.

Bibliography

1. D'Oro et al (1994). Barrier methods of contraception, spermicides, and sexually transmitted diseases: a review. Genitourinary medicine; 70(6): 410–417.
2. Gallo et al (2002). Cervical cap versus diaphragm for contraception. Cochrane Database Systematic Rev;(4):CD003551.

3. Hatcher et al (2009). Contraceptive technology (19th ed.). New York, Ardent Media.

4. Kuyoh et al (2002). Sponge versus diaphragm for contraception. Cochrane Database Syst Rev; (3):CD003172.

5. Macaluso M, Blackwell R, Jamieson DJ, Kulczycki et al (2007). Efficacy of the male latex condom and of the female polyurethane condom as barriers to semen during intercourse: a randomized clinical trial. American journal of epidemiology; 166(1): 88–96.

6. Park K (2015). Preventive and Social Medicine (23rd ed.). Jabalpur: Banarsidas Bhanot Publications.

7. Sahay et al (2015). Failure to Use and Sustain Male Condom Usage: Lessons Learned from a Prospective Study among Men Attending STI Clinic in Pune, India. PloS one; 10(8): e0135071.

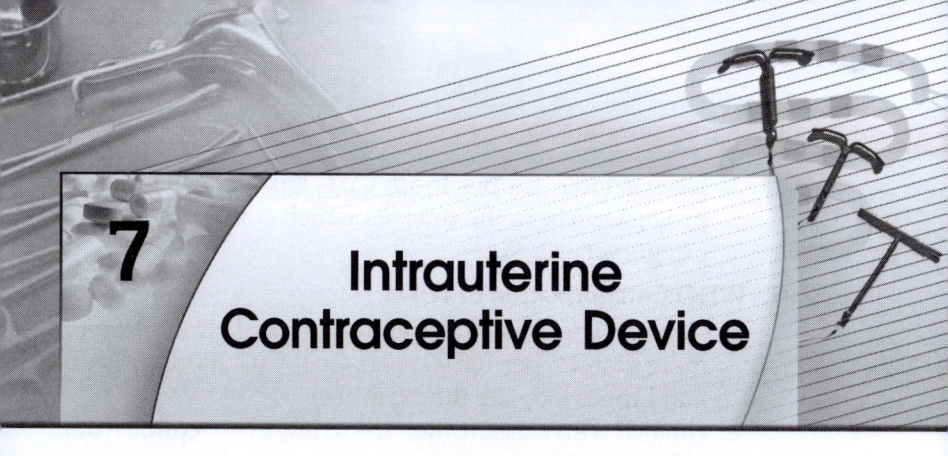

7

Intrauterine Contraceptive Device

Intrauterine contraceptive device is a small device which is often in a 'T' shape containing copper or levonorgesterol and this is inserted into the uterus.

There are several terms used for intrauterine contraception like "intrauterine device, progestin containing device". Intrauterine device is a small device that fits inside the woman's uterus, which cannot be felt or tell it is in there, however, its presence can be checked only by assessing the thread which is felt in the vagina.

History of origination of intrauterine contraceptive device

- Dr Richard Richter from Poland invented an intrauterine ring in 1990.
- Dr Ernst Grafenberg modified the ring for IUD to a coiled metal wire with silk worm gut and silver wire in 1920–1929
- Dr Ota made a ring of gold or gold plated silver in 1934.
- Mr Herbert introduced a stainless steel ring in1949.
- Dr Lazar Margulies invented plastic coil containing barium sulfate in 1960
- Jack Lippies brought Lippes loop made of polyethylene with barium sulfate and nylon thread hanging into the market in 1962
- Mr Zipper and Tatun introduced copper T and Copper 7 in 1969.

Types of Intrauterine Devices

I. **Devices classified based on their shape**

1. *Closed device:* It is a Grafenberg ring and Birnberg bow type of device.

2. *Open devices:* Lippes loop, CuT, Cu7, multiload and progestasert are the devices which comes under this category.

II. WHO Categorization of IUDs

1. *Group I:* This classification has a risk of conception of more than 2% per 100 women. CuT, CuT 200, CuT 200B and Lippes loop are the examples.
2. *Group II:* This classification has a risk of conception from 1–2% per 100 women.
   Examples are Nova T, Cu250, CuT 220C and multiload
3. *Group III:* This classification has a risk of conception below 1% per 100 women. Examples are CuT380A, Cu 375 and LNG IUS.

III. Devices classified based on their content

1. **Nonmedicated (inert)/first generation of IUDs:** It is made-up of polyethylene or other polymers. These are made in different shapes like loops, spirals, coils, rings, and bows. Out of all these, lippies loop is commonly used.

   Lippes loop is double S-shaped plastic material which is nontoxic and made-up of polyethylene material. In order to observe through the X-ray, the device contains a small amount of barium sulfate. It has a tail at the end which is left in the vagina after the insertion, for assurance. This IUD varies in four sizes A, B, C and D.

2. **Medicated (bioactive) devices**
   - **Copper releasing IUDs/second generation of IUDs:** A new approach was tried in the year 1970 with the use of copper metal for anti-fertility. It is smaller in size and easy to fit even in nulliparous women. The IUDs of this generation are CuT 200, mutiload 250, CuT 375 and CuT 380A.
   - **Hormone releasing/third generation of IUDs:** It is mainly T shaped filled with a hormone.
   - **Progestasert:** It is T shaped and contains 38 mg of progesterone. This hormone is released slowly at the rate of 65 µg daily. This can be in situ for 5 yrs.
   - **LNG- 20 (Marena):** It is T-shaped releasing 20 µg of levonorgestrel. It can be *in situ* for 10 yrs.

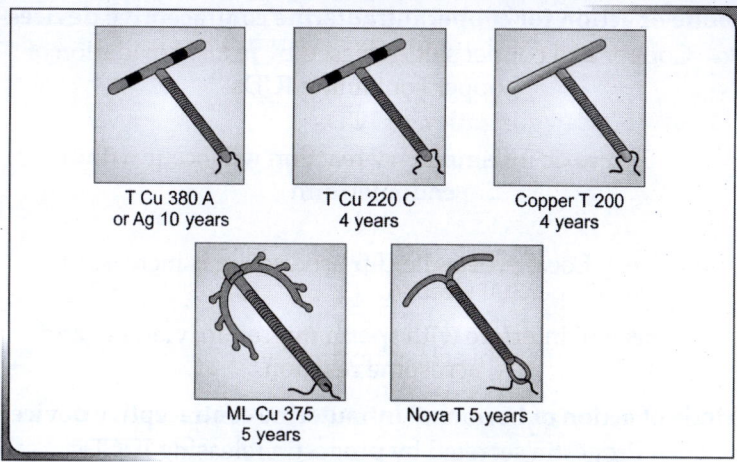

T Cu 380 A
or Ag 10 years

T Cu 220 C
4 years

Copper T 200
4 years

ML Cu 375
5 years

Nova T 5 years

Fig. 7.1 Types of copper T

Selection of Intrauterine Contraceptive Devices

Types of intrauterine contraceptive devices	Conditions which can use the devices
• Estrogen and progestin IUD	Endometrial cancer
• Estrogen-progestin contraceptives and levonorgestrel releasing IUD	Endometriosis and dysmenorrhea
• Copper or levonorgestrel	Safe use as a contraception
• Copper	• Recent breast cancer • Wants to avoid the potential hormonal problems • Would not like to have any interruption in their menstrual cycle • Would like to have uninterrupted contraception for several years • Would like to have emergency contraception • Who need emergency contraception.
• Levonorgestrel	• Treatment of endometrial hyperplasia and cancer • Protects the endometrium • Treating endometriosis • Protecting for endometriosis

Mode of action for copper intrauterine contraceptive devices

Copper and copper salts released by *in utero* oxidation of copper containing IUDs

↓

Cytotoxic inflammatory reaction will occur within endometrium

↓

(e.g. Local prostaglandin production is increased)

↓

This will interfere with sperm migration, viability and acrosome reaction

Mode of action of hormonal intrauterine contraceptive device:

Progestin secreted by progestin releasing IUCDs

↓

It will thickened the cervical mucus

↓

This will create the barrier to sperm penetration into the upper genital tract

↓

- Progestin also causes endometrial decidealization and glandular atrophy, this makes hostile to implantations.
- Progestin also increases expression of glycodin A in endometrial glands which inhibits binding of sperm to the eggs.

Indications

It is useful to women who are:

- Having a desire to have an effective contraception
- Having low risk of acquiring the STDs
- Not having any plans to conceive for at least one year
- Wants to use reversible contraceptives
- Wants to avoid estrogen base methods.

Contraindications

- If there is pregnancy or any suspicious pregnancy
- Any pelvic inflammatory disease (PID)
- Purulent cervicitis

- Puerperal or postabortion sepsis
- Vaginal bleeding which is not considered normal
- Malignancy of the genital tract
- Uterine abnormalities
- Allergic to any of the IUCDs.

Advantages
- Its reversible contraception where the women can conceive if she wishes.
- The different types of intrauterine contraceptive devices have different duration which can be used according to their conveniences.
- It can be in place for 5 years or more than that.
- It can be easily removed by health professionals.
- There is no difficulty in conceiving once the IUCD is removed.
- It does not interfere with the breastfeeding and sexual intercourse.
- Usage of IUCD will not be known to others.
- Third generation IUDs have minimal amount of hormones which do not cause any side effect to women.
- Marina will reduce bleeding which is caused by other disease conditions and also pain

Disadvantages
- Experts are required for insertion
- Nausea and vomiting related to gastro intestinal system may arise
- Complications like infection and perforation of uterus can arise
- Sometimes it can lead to ectopic pregnancy.
- It can cause allergic reaction
- If not fixed properly it can slip down.

Self-care during IUCD insertion

Routine self-care

After each period or at the beginning of each calendar month one should check for the IUD threads.

One should consult a physician if
- There is unusual pain or bleeding
- There is a slip of the IUCD
- There is chance of being pregnant

Relationship with the spouse: IUCDs do not prevent STDs so it is better to have additional protection whose spouse are in sexual relationships with others.

Removal of IUCD
- Any health profession with knowledge regarding IUCD.
- It can cause discomfort for few seconds.
- Alternative contraception must be used before removing the IUD
- The couple should not have any sexual intercourse for at least 7 days before the removal.

Conclusion: IUCDs are contraceptives which can be used by the person under the guidance of health professionals.

Bibliography

1. https://www.uptodate.com/contents/intrauterine-contraception-devices-candidates-and-selection.

8 Hormonal and Chemical Methods

Introduction

One of the important problems in India is ever increasing the rate of population. In 1952 India launched national family planning program to control the birth rate. There are many different birth control methods are used to reduce the fertility. It is the important role of the health care personnel to motivate the community to use various methods of family planning according to their interest. Any method that prevents conception or child birth is known as contraception.

Hormonal contraceptives

1. Oral contraceptives
2. Injectable contraceptive
3. Transdermal patch (implantable contraceptive)
1. Oral contraceptives
   a. Oral pills
      i. Combined pills
      ii. Progesterone—only pill
      iii. Once a month pill

Combined pills

i. Two types of pills are available under the brand name of Mala-N and Mala-D.

Action: Combined pills preventing ovulation of ovum by blocking the secretion of gonadotrophin by pituitary gland. Because of the action of progesterone hormone cervical mucus becomes thick and thus it prevents the entry of sperms and implantation.

ii. Progestogen only pill: Also known as mini pill.

Action: Thickens the cervical mucus, thus it prevents the entry of sperm and implantation of fertilized ovum.

iii. Once a month pill: It is a combined pill of estrogen (long acting) and progesterone.

(Short acting). It is not in use because the chances of pregnancy is high and causes irregular menstrual cycles.

Table 8.1	
Advantages	*Disadvantages*
1. Easy to use	1. If it is taken irregularly, failure rate may increase
2. Does not interfere with coitus	2. Risk of hypertension but it will subside oral pills are discontinued
3. Corrects preexisting menstrual problems	3. User must remember to take pill daily
4. Reduce anemia	4. If it is taken during lactation period, may decrease the quantity of breast milk
5. Reduce risk of pelvic inflammatory disease, colorectal, endometrial, ovarian cancer	5. Increased risk for migraine headache, depression, venous thrombosis and pulmonary embolism lack of appetite, leg cramps
6. Decrease benign breast disease	6. Tenderness in the breast
7. Improves PMS symptoms	7. Weight gain
8. Protects against loss of bone density	8. Excessive pigmentation of the face and forehead
9. Decreased incidence of ectopic preg, uterine fibroids, acne, hirsutism, dysmenorrhea	
10. Very effective and reversible contraception	

Effectiveness: They are the most effective method of contraception, if it is used correctly and consistently the failure rate is 0.1–1 per 100 women. Failure rate depends on missed pills, fear of side effects, delay in starting the next course. If mini pills are used effectively and consistently by lactating women the failure rate is very minimal 0.5% in first year.

Nurses responsibilities

- Complete and history to be collected.
- Provide adequate information about how to use pills.
- Start to take pill on 1st day of menstruation, daily same time preferably before go to bed. In case if she missed pills, she can take the pill whenever she remembers or next day 2 pills together at same regular time.
- If pills are missed for more than 2 days then barrier method can be followed to prevent pregnancy.
- Call for follow up care after 3 months to clear her doubts
- Assess for side effects

2. **Injectable contraceptive:** Depo-Provera is the trade name for an injectable form of a progesterone only contraceptive. It has to be taken once in a 3 months (12 weeks interval) and the dosage is 150 mg. It has to be taken any one day of 5 days of menstrual cycle.

   Action: Suppressing ovulation and the production of FSH and LH by the pituitary gland, thus it increasing the viscosity of cervical mucus and causing endometrial atrophy.

Advantages

1. Safely used during lactation period
2. Reduces excessive bleeding during menstruation and dysmenorrhea
3. Reduces the risks of endometrial and ovarian cancer
4. Reduces the risks of pelvic inflammatory disease, and ectopic pregnancy

Disadvantages

1. Chances of irregular bleeding
2. Amenorrhea
3. Chances of delay in fertility (4–8 months)

Effectiveness

Evidence based practice (EBP): Recent clinical studies raised concern about Depo-Provera reduces the bone mineral density (US Food and Drug Administration, 2015).

4. **Norplant:** It contains 36 mg of levonorgestrel with six flexible closed capsules. From the beginning it releases 85 µg and later 30 µgm per day for five years.

Mode of action: It inhibits ovulation and thus causes atrophy of the endometrium and thickening of the cervical secretion.

Insertion: It is inserted subdermally inner aspect of the non-dominant arm 6–8 cm above the elbow joint under local anesthesia. It is inserted first day of menstrual cycle.

Advantages: Same like injectables.

Other advantages
a. Highly effective and rapidly reversible
b. Benefited for women those who have completed their family
c. Low risk of ectopic pregnancy
d. Best method for women who completed their family and refusing to undergo permanent sterilization

Disadvantages
a. Irregular menstrual bleeding
b. Spotting
c. Expensive
d. Amenorrhoea and irregular bleeding
e. Trained doctor is required for the procedure

Effectiveness: Contraceptive benefits are better than oral contraception and lactation impairment is very less or absent. Iron deficiency anaemia is less, if it is used for long time because of amenorrhoea.

CHEMICAL METHODS

Spermicides: There are four categories
a. Foam—foam tablets, foam aerosols
b. Creams, jellies and pastes—squeezed from a tube
c. Suppositories—inserted manually
d. Soluble films-C—inserted manually

Mode of action: These are chemicals inserted deep into the vagina, near the cervix, before sex. Which attach to the spermatozoa and inhibit oxygen uptake and kill sperms.

Effectiveness

Spermicides are one of the least effective family planning methods, with a 29% chance of pregnancy, and as with other methods effectiveness depends on the user. Risk of pregnancy is greatest when spermicides are not used with every act of sex. In general, spermicides may be an appropriate choice for women who need back-up protection against pregnancy (for instance, if they forget to take their birth control pills). Spermicides should not be used alone as the primary method of birth control. Some concern that there will be teratogenic effects on fetuses.

Advantages

- Safe to use
- Can be used without the help of healthcare personnel
- Increases the vaginal lubrication thus it minimizes vaginal dryness
- There is no hormonal side effect

Disadvantages

- Have high failure rate if it is not used properly.
- It has to be used just before the sexual act and repeated each sex act.
- May cause burning and irritation.

Bibliography

1. Cunningham F (2009). Williams Obstetrics (23rd ed.). McGraw-Hill's Acess Medicine.

2. Mudaliar and Menon's Clinical Obstetrics (2011). (11th ed.). Universities Press (India) Pvt. Ltd.

3. Sharma J (2014). Textbook of Obstetrics (1st ed.). Avichal Publishing Company. ISBN number: 978-81-7739-427-6.

4. Balakrishnan S (2013). Textbook of obstetrics (2nd ed). Paras Medical Publishers, ISBN: 978-81-8191-388-3.

9 Emergency Contraceptive Pills

Emergency contraception is also known as postcoital contraception. It is not a primary contraceptive measure for routine use but it just for backup use.

Indications: Women who had:
- Recent unprotected intercourse
- Sexual assault/rape
- Contraceptive failure or incorrect use, including:
  - Break in a condom or not used correctly.
  - Missed oral contraceptive pills more than three times
  - Displacement, break or tearing of the diaphragm or cervical cap
  - Failure in using withdrawal technique
  - Wrong calculation of the fertile and non-fertile days.
  - IUCD or if hormonal contraceptive implant has expelled.

Different methods of emergency contraceptives

Mainly there are two methods of emergency contraception:
1. Emergency contraceptive pills.
2. Intrauterine device which bears copper.

1. Emergency contraceptive pill:
   The recommended pill according to the WHO is:
   - Levonorgestrel 1.5 mg to be taken within 120 hours or five days of an unprotected sexual intercourse. It must be used only if there is an emergency like unprotected sex, contraceptive failure/misuse and rape. This method is not useful if a pregnancy is established.

- Progestogen-only pill 1.5 mg should be taken as a single dose within five days of unprotected sex. Later levonorgestrel can be taken in 2 doses of 0.75 mg each withinduration of twelve hours.

2. IUCD which bears copper:
   - This IUCD must be inserted within five days of unprotected intercourse. This is an ideal contraception for a woman who would like to continue the contraception for a longer duration.

Mode of action

1. Emergency contraceptive pills work by delaying ovulation
2. Copper IUCD works by inhibiting fertilization

Follow-up

- If pills are vomited out:
  - Within one hour of taking the pills, one has to take it again (advisable to take an antiemetic before taking the pill again).
- Within in 3 hours of taking the pills, then they need to consult a physician for another dose of the pill.
- A pregnancy test is done to confirm conception.

Bibliography

1. Cunningham F (2009). Williams Obstetrics (23rd ed.). McGraw-Hill's Acess Medicine.
2. http://www.uptodate.com/contents/emergency.

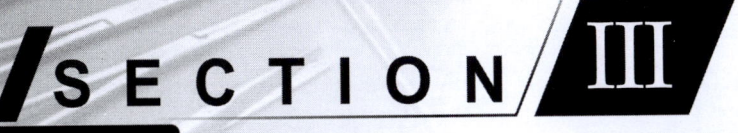

SECTION / III

Instruments

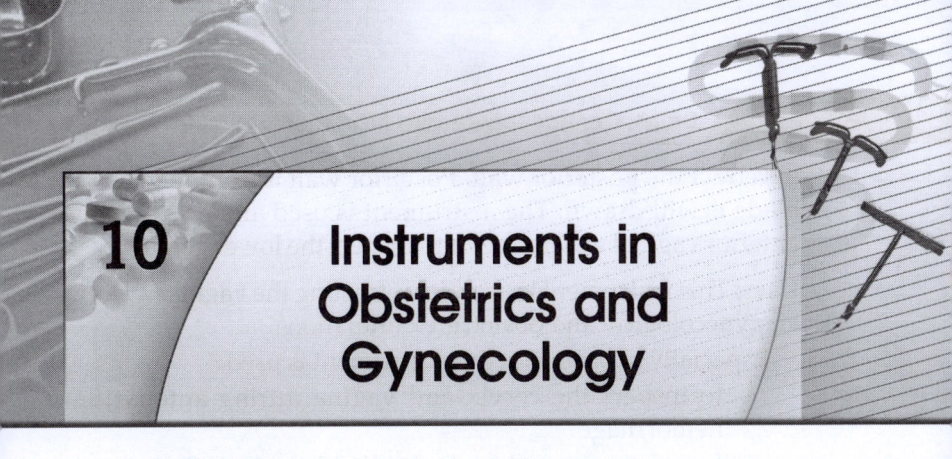

10 Instruments in Obstetrics and Gynecology

Sims' Speculum

A specialized form of vaginal speculum is the weighted speculum, which consists of two blades of unequal breadth, which are introduced into the vagina depending on the space available (narrow blade in nulliparous and wider blade in multiparous women). The blades are smooth and convex as well as at an angle to the shaft and point towards the same side. It has a handle in the centre and one blade at each end is at right angles to the handle (Fig. 10.1). A trough runs along the entire length of the instrument which helps in drainage of secretions by slightly tilting the instrument during inspection of the vagina and vulva.

Technique: First the blade is lubricated with jelly. Labia minora are then separated and the blade inserted with its transverse axis along the long axis of the labia. Blade is then rotated by 90°

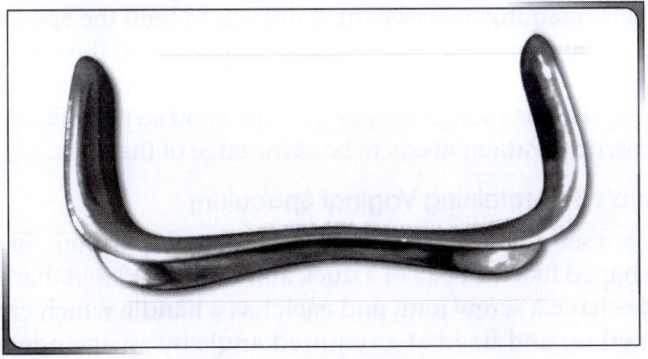

Fig. 10.1: Sims' speculum

to retract the posterior wall. Posterior wall is examined as the blade is withdrawn. The instrument is used along with Sims' anterior vaginal wall retractor to inspect the lower genital tract.

Uses: This instrument is used for retracting the vaginal walls in all gynecological and obstetric examinations.

Especially in obstetrics this instrument is used;

i. to inspect the cervix and vagina during antepartum hemorrhage
ii. for application of Mac Donald's stitches and Shirodkar's operation for cervical incompetence
iii. for cerviprime gel insertion for induction of labor
iv. to inspect the cervix and vagina to detect any injury following delivery
v. to clean the vagina following delivery
vi. while suturing third degree perineal tear and cervical tears
vii. for examining and packing the uterus during postpartum hemorrhage
viii. Intrauterine contraceptive device insertion, follow-up and removal

In Gynecological cases this instrument used;

i. while taking cervical biopsy and cytology
ii. during vaginal hysterectomy
iii. for removal of polyps.

The main advantage of this instrument is it gives a better field of view than Cusco's bivalve self-retaining speculum. Since it is not self-retaining an assistant is needed to hold the speculum during the procedure and for good inspection of the posterior vaginal wall; anterior vaginal wall retractor is also needed for proper visualization. It moves with the hand so not suitable for colposcopy. Patient needs to be at the edge of the table.

Cusco's Self-retaining Vaginal Speculum

This is a self-retaining double bladed vaginal speculum. Blades are shaped like the beak of a duck and are hinged together. The blades have a screw joint and each has a handle which can be opened up and fixed at a required angle by an arrangement which is adjustable (Fig. 10.2). They are available in various sizes.

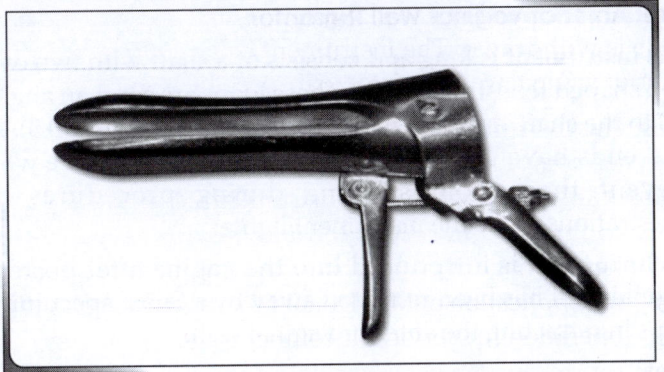

Fig. 10.2: Cusco's self-retaining vaginal speculum

Technique: The blades are closed and then introduced in an anteroposterior direction and rotated by 90° may cause minimal discomfort to the patient. The fixation screw is then tightened depending on amount of exposure needed.

Uses: It is an ideal instrument for operating the cervix. It is used in out-patient department for routine examinations and to perform minor procedures and also in minor operations, not requiring excessive retraction of vaginal walls. For example:

i. To view vagina and cervix
ii. To obtain cultural material from cervix
iii. To obtain biopsy material (cervical biopsy)
iv. To apply medication
v. To take Pap's smear
vi. To cauterise a lesion
vii. Intrauterine contraceptive device (IUCD) insertion
viii. Colposcopy
ix. Cautery and cryosurgery of cervical lesions

The advantage of this instrument is, no assistant is required during procedure and it causes lesser discomfort to the patient and gives a very good view of cervix but limited field of vision is available and covers both the anterior and the posterior vaginal walls, decreased maneuverability and less space to perform dilatation and curettage.

Sims' Anterior Vaginal Wall Retractor

This instrument is long and consists of a shaft with two oval/ loop shaped fenestrated ends. These loops are set at an angle of 150 to the shaft, and face in opposite directions (Fig. 10.3). The oval ends have transverse serrations on the surface which prevent them from slipping during procedures and fenestrations make the instrument lighter.

Technique: It is introduced into the vagina after posterior vaginal wall has been retracted away by a Sims' speculum. It helps in retracting the anterior vaginal wall.

Uses:

i. It is used in all gynaecological and obstetrical operations requiring visualization of the cervix and anterior vaginal wall.

ii. It can also be used as a blunt curette in cases of post-partum hemorrhage just after the delivery.

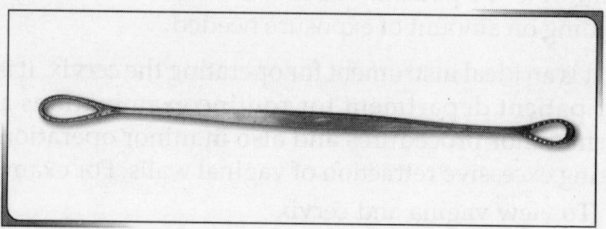

Fig. 10.3: Sims' anterior vaginal wall retractor

Teale's Vulsellum Forceps

This instrument is long consisting of two blades with sharp multiple teeth which can interlock, and it consists of a joint, shank, handles and a lock (Fig. 10.4). The blades are curved from the side and there is a distance between the blades which prevents crushing of the tissue held in between. The sharp tooth provides a firm grip and at the same time causes minimum injury. The curve helps by not blocking the field of vision and causing lesser discomfort to the patient. The instrument helps in steadying the cervix.

Technique: The cervix is visualized after retracting the posterior wall with Sims' speculum and anterior vaginal wall with anterior vaginal wall retractor. The anterior lip of the cervix is

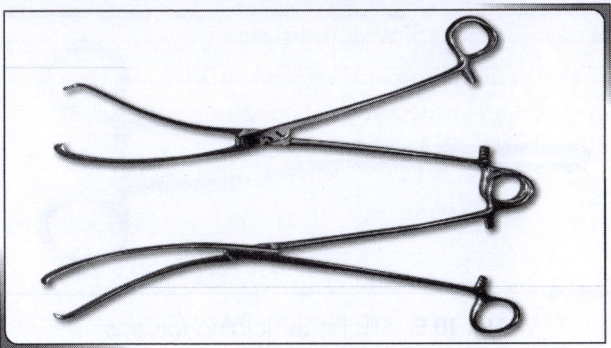

Fig. 10.4: Teale's vulsellum forceps

then grasped with teeth of the blades and instrument is then locked after obtaining a firm grip of the cervix. The curve of the instrument should face upwards so that it will not block the field of vision.

Uses: It is used to;
- catch hold the anterior lip of cervix in operations on cervix and uterus
- hold the cervix during dilatation
- hold the cervix in vaginal hysterectomy
- hold the fibroids during operation
- test the mobility of the cervix and laxity of its ligaments in case of prolapse.

Allis Tissue Holding Forceps

It is a straight instrument with two blades, and a handle with lock and finger bows (Fig. 10.5). The blades have distance in between and come close together only at the tips and are toothed. The lock and toothed blades provide a firm grip. The distance between the blades prevents crushing of the tissue held in between. The teeth are multiple and fine which cause least trauma to the soft tissues. This instrument is available both in small sizes and large sizes.

Uses:
  i. To hold the thin but tough structures like skin and rectus sheath during opening and closure of abdominal surgeries

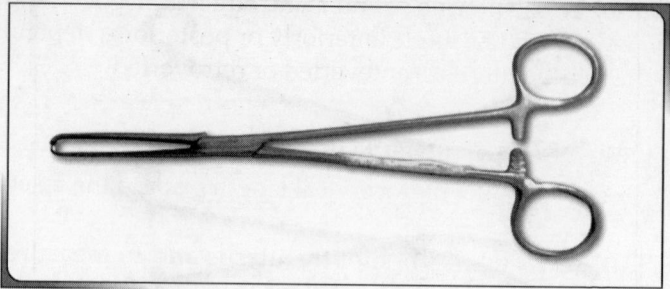

Fig. 10.5: Allis tissue holding forceps

   ii. To hold the cervix in dilatation and curettage, hystero-salphingo graphy, etc.

 iii. In lower segment cesarean section for holding the edges of the uterine incision

 iv. To hold the apex of any wound which is being repaired, e.g. episiotomy, perineal tear, etc.

  v. It can be used as a towel clip

 vi. To hold the peanut swabs to control oozing in the operation field.

Simpson's Uterine Sound

The instrument is 12 inches (30 cm) long and is marked in inches or centimetres. It has an angled distal end, a shaft and a handle (Fig. 10.6). The instrument is Olive tipped (to avoid perforation). It is bent at an angle of 1500 at a distance of 6.5 cm from its tip, i.e. at a distance equal to the normal uterocervical length. It has markings on it for measurements.

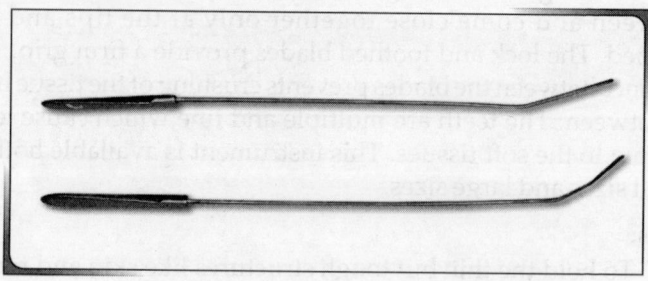

Fig. 10.6: Simpson's uterine sound

Technique: The uterine sound is introduced in a pen holding manner keeping the angle anteriorly or posteriorly depending on whether the uterus is anteverted or retroverted.

Uses:
   i. It acts as a first dilator of the cervical canal.
  ii. To measure the uterocervical length prior to the insertion of an IUCD.
 iii. To know the position of the uterus and to measure the length of the uterine cavity prior to the dilatation of the cervix in dilatation and evacuation operation.
  iv. It is also used to differentiate between the inversion of the uterus and uterine polyp.
   v. It is used to feel for any pathology inside such as fibroid uterus, septate/bicornuated uterus or adhesions or uterine synechiae.

The main disadvantage of this instrument is, it can cause perforation of the uterus if the direction of the uterus or its size is misjudged and if the sound is introduced in the wrong direction.

Hegar's Dilators

These instruments are sinuously curved double ended instruments and have conical tips (Fig. 10.7). The tips are angled to the shaft and point in opposite directions. They are available in gradually increasing sizes. The minimum size is ½ and

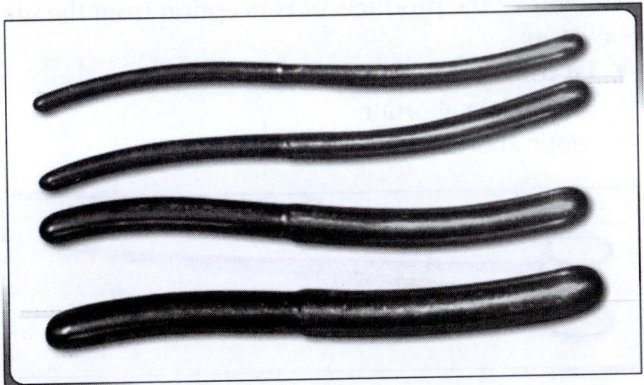

Fig. 10.7: Hegar's dilators

maximum size is 11/12. The number represents the diameter in millimetres. Two sizes are available in one double ended dilator with a difference of 1 mm in their diameter. Both the sides are used with the lower number first.

Uses:

i. It is used in dilatation of the cervical canal prior to evacuation operation such as incomplete abortion, suction evacuation and medical termination of pregnancy by dilatation and evacuation (D and E).

ii. Dilatation of the cervix is required in many obstetrical and gynecological cases such as; tubal insufflation test and hystero salphingography (HSG), intrauterine contraceptive device (IUCD) insertion, prior to intracavity radiation, etc.

iii. Smaller sizes are used as urethral dilators.

Heywood Smith's Ovum Forceps

It is a long instrument with two blades—spoon shaped, blunt with fenestrated ends and which just touch each other when the forceps is closed so that anything held in the blades is firmly caught but not crushed at its base (Fig. 10.8). It has no lock, so it minimizes damage to any structure which may be accidentally held in between the blades. This forceps is available in varying sizes of blades used according to the necessity. The fenestrations allow part of the tissue to bulge out so that the grip is secure.

Uses:

i. To remove the products of conception from the uterine cavity in:
   • 1st trimester pregnancy termination
   • Incomplete abortion
   • Septic abortion

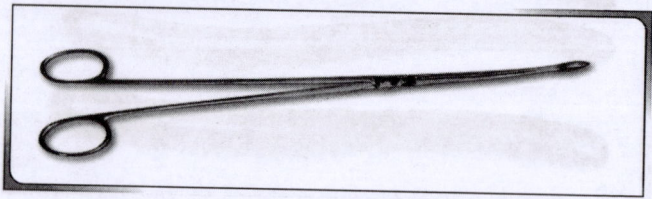

Fig. 10.8: Heywood Smith's ovum forceps

ii. To explore the uterine for placental bits and membranes in postpartum hemorrhage (PPH)

iii. To remove foreign bodies from the uterus (e.g. in case of septic abortion)

iv. To twist the pedunculated uterine or cervical polyp.

Uterine Curette

It is long, double ended instrument. It has a central shaft and terminal ends have small oval loops which are angled to the shaft (Fig. 10.9). The two loops are angled in opposite directions. The loops at both ends are sharp, one end may be less sharp/blunt than the other. The curette comes in different sizes. The size of the loop varies between 6 to 10 mm. The sharp end has smaller sized loop while blunt end has a larger loop. Only blunt curette is used in obstetrics, since the uterus is soft and can be easily perforated by a sharp curette.

Uses: Blunt edge of the instrument is used for the curetting the uterus after cervical dilatation in different obstetric operations such as:

- Incomplete abortion, by dilatation and curettage
- Dilatation and evacuation operation
- Medical termination of pregnancy by ovum forceps
- Check curettage after vesicular mole evacuation
- Septic abortion.

Sharp edge of the instrument is used in gynaecological indications such as:

- Dysfunctional uterine bleeding (DUB)
- For fractional curettage in cases of cancer endometrium and
- To assess the extent of uterine involvement in cervix carcinoma
- To diagnose the causes of postmenopausal bleeding,

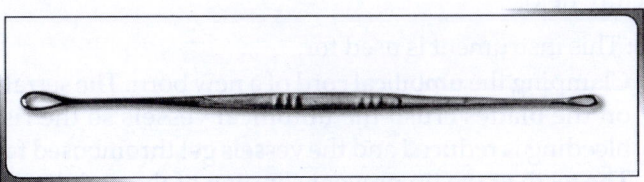

Fig. 10.9: Uterine curette

- To break the adhesions in case of Asherman's syndrome (AS) or Fritsch syndrome is a condition characterized by adhesions and/or fibrosis of the endometrium most often associated with dilation and curettage of the intrauterine cavity).

The disadvantage of this instrument is, overexcited curettage can result in Asherman's syndrome leading to amenorrhea, infertility, haemorrhage and cervical injuries.

Uterine Polyp Forceps

This instrument has slender blades ending in flat end ovals (Fig. 10.10). The blades have fenestrations and transverse serrations. The instrument has a joint, handles with finger grips and a lock forgripping the uterine polyps firmly.

Uses: For removal of endometrial polyps.

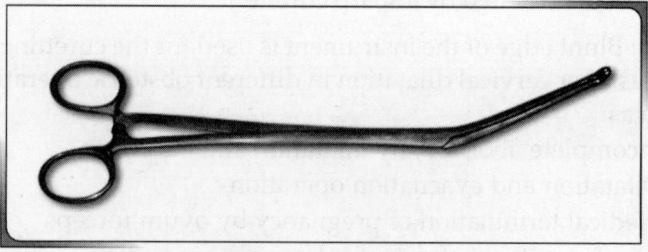

Fig. 10.10: Uterine polyp forceps

Umbilical Cord Clamp/Kocher's Clamp

This instrument is curved/straight consisting of two blades, a joint, a lock and handle with finger grips (Fig. 10.11). The blades are specially designed to serve the function as efficient hemostats. They have transverse serrations on the inner aspect and are toothed. They together provide very firm grip of the structure held.

Uses: This instrument is used for:
  i. Clamping the umbilical cord of a new born: The serrations on the blades crush the umbilical vessels so the risk of bleeding is reduced and the vessels get thrombosed faster. The teeth at the tip prevent slipping of the umbilical cord through the clamp.

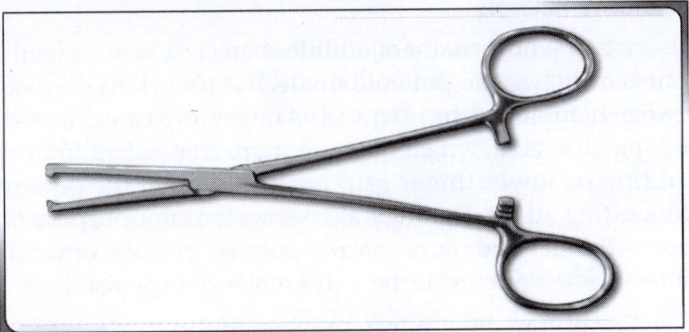

Fig. 10.11: Umbilical cord clamp/Kocher's clamp

  ii. Performing artificial low rupture of membranes (ARM) during labor.
 iii. Holding tough structures like, rectus sheet while closing the abdomen as in a Pfannenstiel incision.

Sponge Holding Forceps

This instrument is 22.5 cm long has ring shaped tips, serrated or smoothed, straight or curved (Fig. 10.12).

Uses: This instrument is used for:
   i. Swabbing out cavities like vagina or the pelvic cavity
  ii. Antiseptic painting of skin, vulva and vagina
 iii. Applying pressure over bleeding points
  iv. Grasping a cervix in obstetric practice
   v. Temporarily clamping of the infundibular pelvic ligament
  vi. Grasping a lip of a torn cervix.

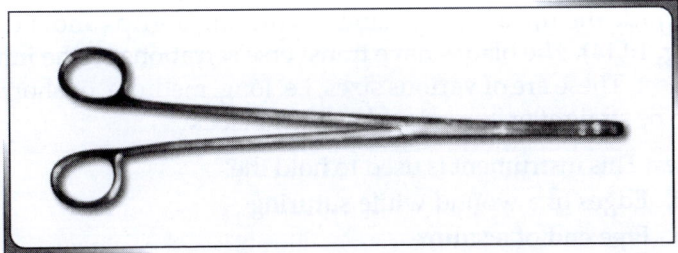

Fig. 10.12: Spongeholding forceps

Episiotomy Scissors

This instrument is made of stainless steel. It is sterilized by immersing in lysol or glutaraldehyde. It is 16 cm long. Its blades are angled on side at the joint and its finger grips are directed in the same direction, which makes it more convenient to use by avoiding its lower finger grip butting against the patient's buttocks (Fig. 10.13). The angle also serves the same purpose. One blade is thinner and more sharply pointed than the other. The thinner blade is put inside the vulva while giving episiotomy.

Uses: For giving episiotomy (perineotomy) during the 2nd stage of labor to enlarge the introitus to facilitate easy and safe delivery of the fetus and to minimize the overstretching and rupture of the perineal muscles.

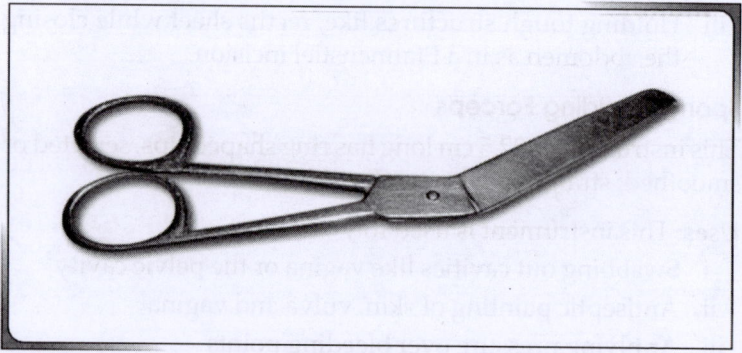

Fig. 10.13: Episiotomy scissors

Artery Forceps

They have thick and strong two blades tapering gradually towards the tip, a joint, a handle with finger grips and a lock (Fig. 10.14). The blades have transverse serrations on the inner aspect. These are of various sizes, i.e. long, medium, or short. It can be straight or curved with a Ratchet lock.

Uses: This instrument is used to hold the:
  i. Edges of a wound while suturing
 ii. Free end of a suture
iii. Bleeders for ligating and cauterization

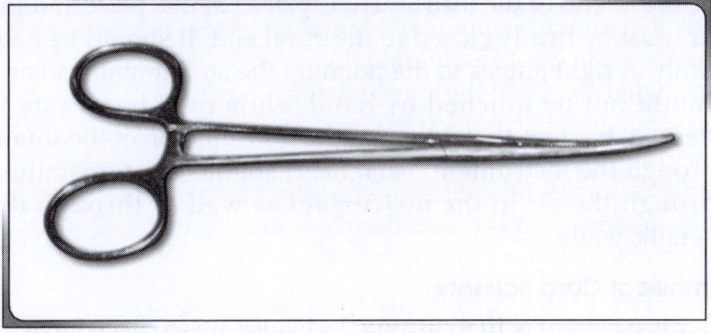

Fig. 10.14: Artery forceps

Pinard's Fetal Stethoscope

Pinard's fetal stethoscope is an instrument designed to hear the fetal heart sounds during the antenatal period from 24 weeks onwards and during labor. Fetal stethoscope is 40 cm long, funnel shaped, with the broad flat disc attached at narrow end and has opening in the center for conduction of sound (Fig. 10.15). Material used may be plastic, aluminium or rarely wood. The metal stethoscope is cheaper and easier to make. However, its shape alters readily on falling. It is also cold to touch in the winter. Wooden stethoscope is made narrower. Its shape does not change and it does not feel cold to touch in winter.

Method of use: The patient is put in supine position with 15° left lateral tilt. The position of the anterior shoulder is determined by palpation. Standing on the patient's right side

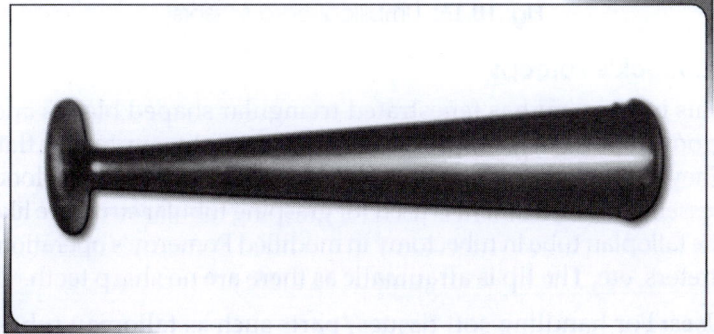

Fig. 10.15: Pinard's fetal stethoscope

the broad end of the instrument is placed at this place and the ear must be firmly closed to the aural end. It should be held firmly at right angles to the point on the abdominal wall and should not be touched by hand while fetal heart rate is checked, because that dampens the transmission of the sound through the instrument. Fetal heart sounds are transmitted through the air in the instrument as well as through the metallic walls.

Umbilical Cord Scissors

This instrument is 10.5 cm long. Its blades are so curved that on closing they meet only at their tips, leaving a gap in between which ensures the firm grip on umbilical cord when the cord is being cut (Fig. 10.16). With an ordinary scissors the cord tends to slip away from the scissors because it contains Wharton's jelly and is covered by smooth amniotic membrane.

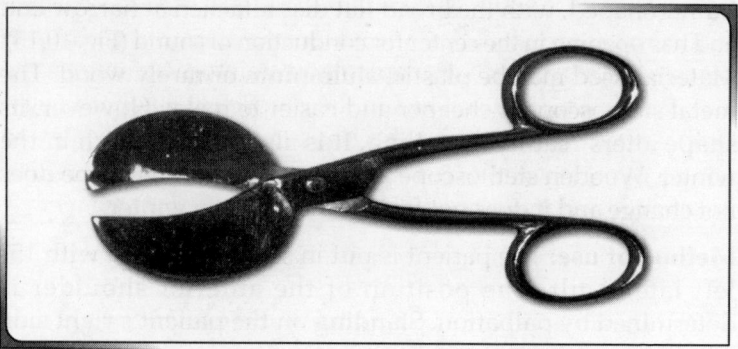

Fig. 10.16: Umbilical cord scissors

Babcock's Forceps

This instrument has fenestrated triangular shaped blades and grooved jaws (Fig. 10.17). They can be straight, curved on flat. They ensure firm grip without damaging or crushing the blood vessels. This instrument is used for grasping tubular structure like the fallopian tube in tubectomy in modified Pomeroy's operation, ureters, etc. The tip is atraumatic as there are no sharp teeth.

Uses: For handling soft tissues/parts such as fallopian tubes, intestine, ureter, appendix, etc.

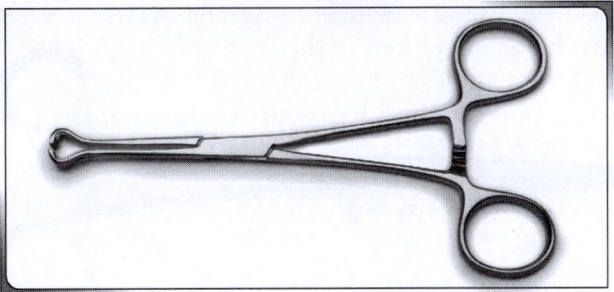

Fig. 10.17: Babcock's forceps

Ayre's Spatula

This spatula is made of wood or plastic and is shaped to fit the shape of the cervix (Fig. 10.18). The tip of the spatula is inserted to the cervical canal and the spatula is rotated in complete circle to take the cervical smear. The smear/scrapings are spread on a slide and immediately dropped in a mixture of equal parts of 95% alcohol and ether. The smear is then stained with Papanicolaou method. (Papanicolaou stain or Pap stain is the most important stain utilized in the practice of cytopathology. It is a polychromatic stain containing multiple dyes to differentially stain various components of the cells. This technique was developed by George Papanicolaou, the father of cytopathology.)

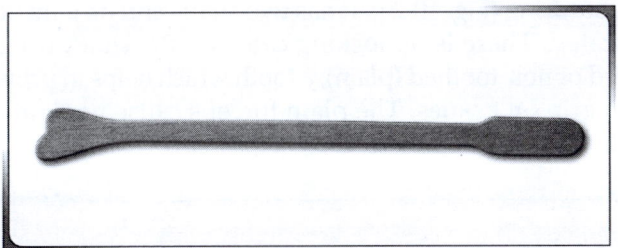

Fig. 10.18: Ayre's spatula

Needle Holder

This instrument is used to hold curved needles. The shape is similar to of artery forceps but the blades are smaller and the serrations on the inner surface are crisscrossed with one blade

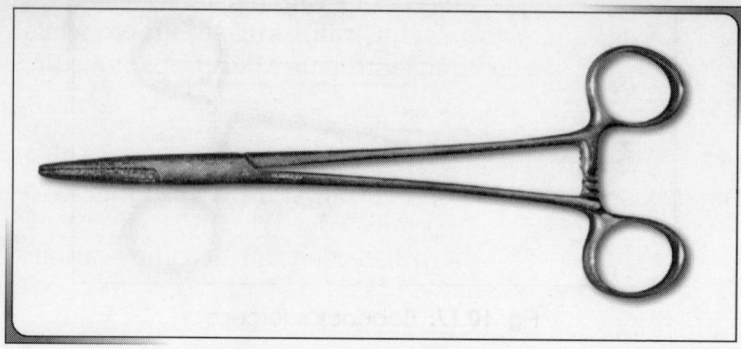

Fig. 10.19: Needle holder

having a longitudinal groove to prevent slipping and turning of the needle (Fig. 10.19). It has a shaft with the rings for thumb and finger with Ratchet lock for a firm grip. The instrument is available both in small and large sizes.

Types available are straight type and curved. Straight type is also called Blalock's type and curved type is also called Kilner's type which is used in cavities as the curved needle does not obstruct the view of the operating field.

Dissecting Forceps

This is also known as thumb forceps. It is a two-armed instrument used for holding tissues either during dissection or while suturing (Fig. 10.20). It has two shafts and no joint, the tip is serrated. There is no locking catch on the shaft. It may be toothed or non-toothed (plain), a tooth which helps in providing a firm grip on tissues. The plain forceps cause no damage to tissues whereas toothed forceps helps in providing a firm grip.

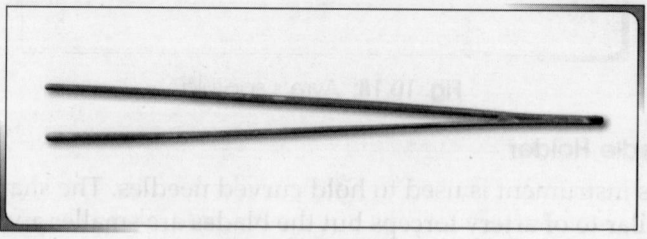

Fig. 10.20: Dissecting forceps

Uses: The toothed type is used for steadying tough structures like the edges of the vaginal vault, wall, rectus sheath, etc. while plain is used for soft and friable structures like the peritoneum, uterine edges, etc.

Scissors

Scissors can be long or short, strong or fine, blunt or sharp pointed, straight or curved on the edge (Fig. 10.21). These are used for blunt as well as sharp dissection and for cutting various pedicles and sutures.

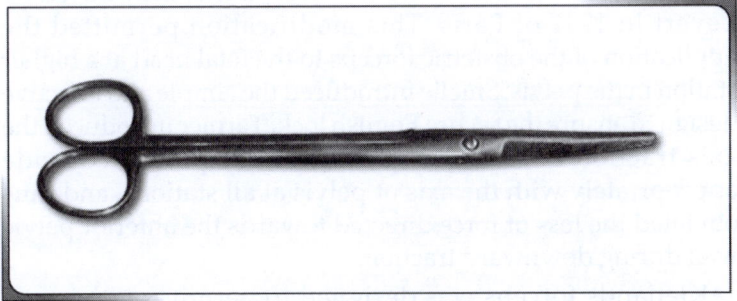

Fig. 10.21: Scissors

Obstetric Forceps and Vacuum Device

These instruments are mainly used for operative vaginal delivery also termed instrumental or assisted vaginal birth. Operative vaginal delivery refers to a delivery in which the operator uses forceps or a vacuum device to assist the mother in transitioning the fetus to extrauterine life. The instrument is applied to the fetal head and then the operator uses traction to extract the fetus, typically during a contraction while the mother is pushing.

It is commonly used to expedite birth for the benefit of either mother or baby or both. It is sometimes associated with significant complications for both mother and baby. The choice of instrument may be influenced by clinical circumstances, operator choice, and availability of specific instruments.

The main aim of this operative vaginal delivery is to achieve a vaginal birth and avoiding significant morbidity for mother and baby.

Obstetric Forceps

These are pair of instruments specially designed to assist extraction of the fetal head and thereby accomplish the delivery of the fetus.

Obstetric forceps were introduced in the 17th century by the Chamberlain family, England and have been modified and adapted in various forms. The credit for designing of the precursor of modern forceps goes to Peter Chamberlain (about 1600 AD) of England.

Pelvic curve in the obstetrics forceps was introduced by Levert in 1747 of Paris. This modification permitted the application of the obstetric forceps to the fetal head at a higher station in the pelvis. Smelie introduced the simple and effective design to ensure the secure English lock. Tarnier introduced the axis traction device. This permitted the pull to coincide appropriately with the axis of pelvis at all stations, and thus obviated the loss of force directed towards the anterior pelvic wall during downward traction.

Kiellands forceps was designed to permit rotation and extraction of the baby. In India, the mid-cavity forceps was modified by K.N. Das.

Varieties of obstetric forceps:
- Long curved forceps with or without axis traction device
- Short curved forceps
- Kiellands forceps.

Long Curved Obstetric Forceps

This instrument is relatively heavy and is about 37 cm (15″) long. The distance in between the tips is 2.5 cm and widest diameter between the blades is 9 cm.

These instruments basically consist of two crossing branches. Each branch has four components: blades, shank, lock, and handle with or without screw (Fig. 10.22).

The blade is fenestrated to facilitate a good grip of the fetal head. There is usually a slot in the lower part of the fenestrum of the blade to allow the upper end of the axis traction rod to be fitted.

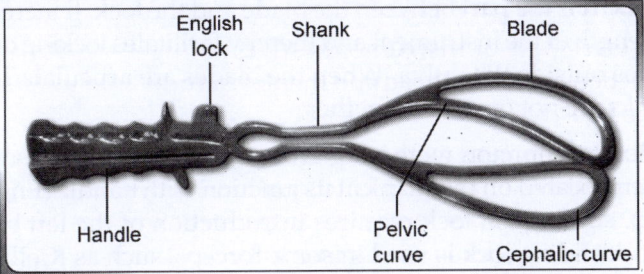

Fig. 10.22: Long curved obstetric forceps

The blade has got two curves namely the pelvic curve and the cephalic curve.

1. **Pelvic curve:** Corresponds more or less to the axis of the birth canal (curve of Carus)
2. **Cephalic curve:** Conforms to the shape of the fetal head which when articulated grasps the fetal head without compression.

The blades are connected to the handles by the shanks.

Identification of the Blades

When articulated: Place the instrument in front of the pelvis with the tip of the blades pointing upwards and the concave side of the pelvic curve forwards (Fig. 10.23).

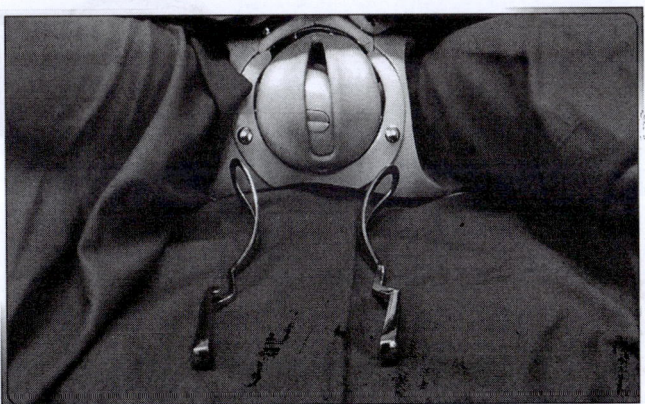

Fig. 10.23: The blade which corresponds to the left of the maternal pelvis is the left blade and to the right side is the right blade

Shank: It is the part between the blade and the lock. It increases the length of the instrument and thereby facilitates locking of the blades outside the vulva. When the blades are articulated, the shanks are not opposed together.

Lock: The common method of articulation consists of a socket system located on the shank at its junction with handle (English lock). An English lock requires introduction of the left blade first. A sliding lock is used in some forceps, such as Kiellands forceps (Fig. 6.26).

Handle: The handles are opposed when blades are articulated. There is a finger guard for placing the finger during traction.

A screw may be attached usually at the end or at the base of one blade (commonly left). It helps to keep the blades in position.

Axis Traction Device

It can be applied with advantage in mid forceps operation, especially following manual rotation of the head. It provides traction in the current axis of the pelvic curve and as such, less force is necessary to deliver the head. It consists of traction rods and traction handle (Fig. 10.24).

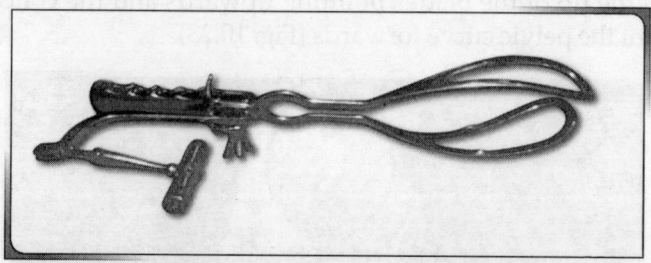

Fig. 10.24: Long forceps with axis traction device

Wrigley's Short Curved Obstetric Forceps

It is a small light forceps about one-third the weight of the long obstetric forceps. The length is only 11 inches which is due to reduction in the length of the shanks and the handles. The maximum distance between the closed blades is 3 inches and between tips is 1 inch (Fig. 10.25). It has an English type fixed lock.

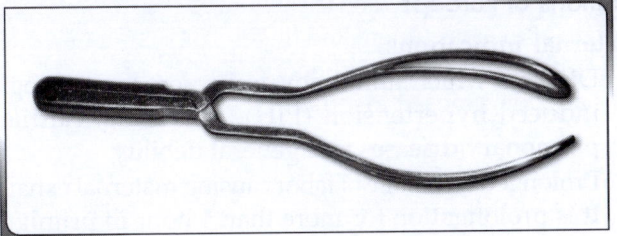

Fig. 10.25: Wrigley's short curved obstetric forceps

Uses: It is used as an outlet forceps when the fetal head is at or below + 2 station.

Kielland's Forceps

This instrument is long straight obstetric forceps without any axis traction device. One small knob on each blade is directed towards the occiput of the fetal head (Fig. 10.26). The forceps have a cephalic curve and a negligible pelvic curve. The length is 15.5 inches and the maximum distance between the blades is variable as it has a sliding lock. The lock is sliding type with a claw handle and fish tail end. The advantage of the sliding lock is that it can deliver the head by asynclitism. It is long heavy forceps and is associated with severe maternal injuries.

Uses: These forceps is now obsolete. It was earlier used for high forceps operations with the biparietal diameter lying above the pelvic brim but now this operation has been discarded.

It can be used for rotation in extraction of head in persistent occipitoposterior position or deep transverse arrest. The absence of a well-defined pelvic curve makes it a useful instrument for rotating the head.

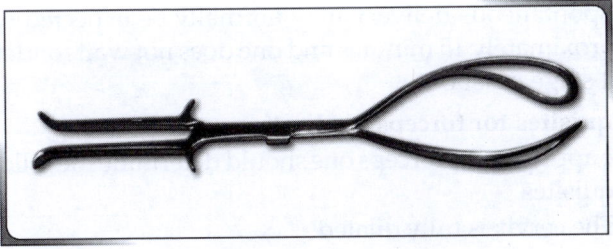

Fig. 10.26: Kielland's forceps

Indications of Forceps

1. Maternal indications

i. Diseases which limits physical reserve, e.g. pregnancy induced hypertension (PIH), eclampsia, cardiac and pulmonary diseases and general debility.

ii. Prolonged 2nd stage of labor causing maternal exhaustion. It is prolongation for more than 1 hour in primigravida or 30 minutes in multipara. This may be due to Inertia and poor voluntary bearing down and large fetus.

iii. Used for malposition's like persistent occipitoposterior position and deep transverse arrest.

iv. Failure to bear down during the 2nd stage of labor due to regional block anesthesia, excessive sedation or psychiatric disturbances.

2. Fetal indications

i. Fetal distress

ii. Cord prolapse

iii. Delay of delivery of after coming head in breech presentation

iv. Certain malpresentations—selected cases of face presentation

3. Prophylactic forceps

It is an expression to describe forceps before fetal and maternal distress or prolongation of 2nd stage. In some multiparous women, rigid perineum at vaginal introitus offers a marked resistance to the fetal head in the 2nd stage, which in turn can lead to fetal brain damage and maternal perineal floor nerve damage. To avoid this Dee Lee (1920) recommended the prophylactic forceps operation or low elective forceps so spontaneous delivery may normally be expected within approximately 15 minutes and one does not wait for delayed 2nd stage of labor.

Prerequisites for forceps application

Before applying the forceps one should determine the following prerequisites

i. The cervix is fully dilated.

ii. The membranes are ruptured.

iii. The fetal head must be engaged, flexed and preferably well-rotated.

iv. Uterus must be contracting.

v. The bladder must be empty.

vi. There must be no obvious cephalopelvic disproportion.

vii. If fetal presentation or position is uncertain, intrapartum ultrasound examination should be performed, as it is more accurate than digital examination.

viii. The fetal size has been estimated and clinical pelvimetry indicates adequate mid and outlet pelvic dimensions, and no obstructions or contractures exist.

ix. Maternal anesthesia is satisfactory. Neuraxial anesthesia provides more effective analgesia than pudendal block.

x. Maternal bladder is empty.

xi. The option of performing an immediate cesarean delivery is available if complications arise. Personnel for neonatal resuscitation are available, if needed.

Types of the application:

i. *Cephalic application:* The blades are applied along the sides of the head grasping the biparietal diameter in between the widest part of the blades. The long axis of the blades corresponds to the occipitomental plane of the fetal head. It is the ideal method of application as it has a negligible compression effect on the fetal head.

ii. *Pelvic application:* When the blades of the forceps are applied on the lateral pelvic walls ignoring the position of the head, it is called pelvic application. If the head remains unrotated this type of application puts serious compression on the cranium and that must be avoided.

Application

Forceps—appropriately applied forceps grasp the occiput anterior (OA) fetal head such that:

- The long axis of the blades corresponds to the occipitomental diameter.
- The tips of the blades lie over the cheeks of the fetus.
- The blades are equidistant from the sagittal suture, which should bisect a horizontal plane through the shanks.

- The posterior fontanelle should be one finger breadth anterior to this plane.
- Fenestrated blades should admit no more than one finger breadth between the heel of the fenestration and the fetal head.
- No maternal tissue should be grasped.
- Rotation, when needed, is performed between contractions. These deliveries are more difficult and associated with a higher risk of maternal and fetal complications than simple traction applied to the non- or minimally rotated vertex.
- To reduce the risk of laceration, forceps are disarticulated and removed when expulsion is certain, but before the widest diameter of the fetal head passes through the introitus. The vertex can then be delivered with no or minimal maternal assistance.

Low Forceps Operation

Preliminaries

- General or local anesthesia is used or in some cases operational intravenous diazepam is used.
- The patient is placed in lithotomy position.
- Full surgical asepsis is taken.
- Surgeon has to wear sterile mask, gown and gloves.
- Vulva and vagina are to be washed with antiseptic solution.
- Cervix is cleaned with povidine iodine solution.
- The perineum is to be draped by sterile towel and the legs with leggings.
- Bladder should be emptied.
- Vaginal examination should be done: to assess the state of the cervix, membranous status, presentation, position of the head and assessment of pelvic outlet.
- Episiotomy is usually done during the traction when the perineum becomes bulged and thinned out by the advancing head.

The operation consists of the following steps:

   i. Identification and application of the blade

   ii. Locking of the blade

  iii. Traction

  iv. Removal of the blade.

Step i. Identification and application of the blade

- The identification should be done after the articulation of the blade, the left or lower blade is introduced first.
- The four fingers of the semi-supinated right hand are inserted along the left lateral vaginal wall (Fig. 10.27).
- The palmar surface of the fingers rest against the side of the head.
- The fingers guide the blade during the application and this helps protecting the vaginal wall.
- The handle of the left blade is taken lightly by three fingers to the left-hand index, middle, and the thumb in a pen holding manner and is held vertically almost parallel to the right inguinal ligament.
- The fenestrated portion of the blades placed on the right palm with tip pointing upwards. The right thumb is placed at the junction of the blade and the shank (heel).
- The blade is introduced between the gliding internal fingers and the fetal head, manipulated by the thumb.
- As the blade is pushed up, the handle is carried downwards and backwards, traversing the wide arc of a circle towards the left until the shank lies straight on the perineum thus gently introducing the blade.
- No assistant is usually required to hold the handle in low forceps operation. When correctly applied, the blade should be over the parietal eminence, the shank should be in contact with the perineum and the superior surface of the handle should be directed upwards.

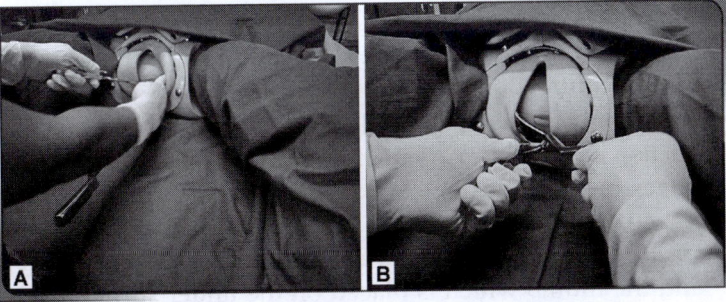

Fig. 10.27: Application of the blade

Application of the right blade
- The two fingers of the right hand can introduce into the right lateral wall of the vagina along side the baby's head.
- The right blade is introduced in the same manner as with left one but holding it with right hand.

Step ii. Locking of the blades
- When correctly applied, the blade should be manipulated with ease.
- Minor difficulty in locking can be corrected by depressing the handles on the perineum (Fig. 10.28).
- In case of major difficulty, the blades are to be removed. The causes are then sought for and the blades are to be reinserted.

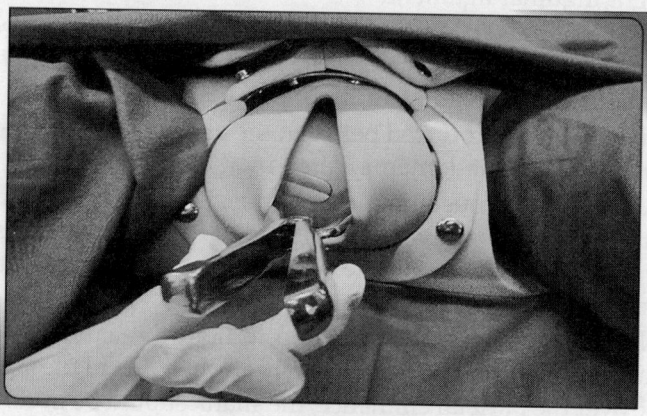

Fig. 10.28: Locking of the blades

Steps iii and iv. Traction and removal of the blades
Principles
- Steady but intermittent traction should be given if possible during contraction.
- Gripping of the articulated forceps during traction. The traction is given by gripping the handle by placing the middle finger in between the shanks with the ring and the index finger on either side of the finger-guard. During the final traction the four fingers are placed in between the shank and the thumb which is placed on the under surface of the handles and necessary force is exerted.

- Direction of the pull corresponds to the axis of the birth canal. In low forceps depending on the station of the head the direction of pull downwards and backwards until the head comes to the perineum. The pull is then directed horizontally straight towards the operator till the head is almost crowned. The direction of the head is then upwards and forwards towards the mother's abdomen to deliver the head by extension. The blades are removed one after the other with the right one first (Fig. 10.29).
- Following the delivery of the head the usual procedure is followed as in a normal delivery.

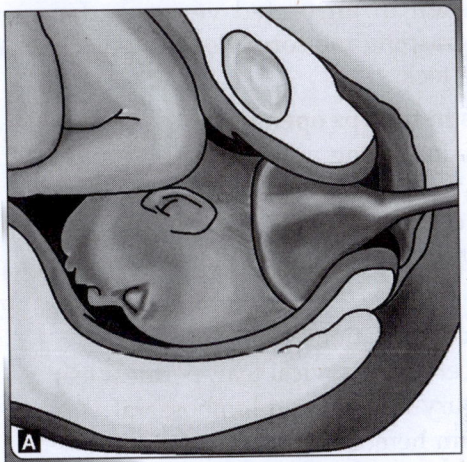

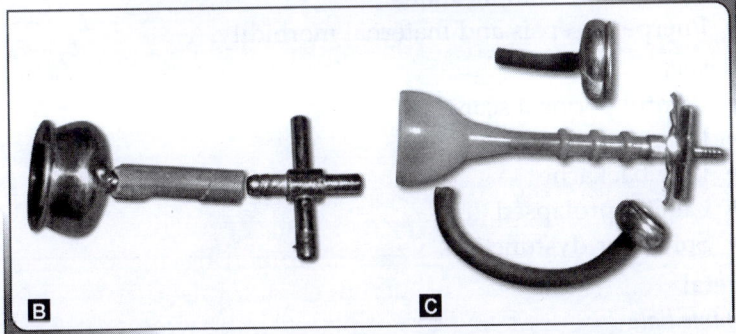

Fig. 10.29: (A) Extraction and delivery of fetal head applying ventouse or vacuum extractor; (B) Ventouse or vacuum extractor; (C) Silastic cup

Outlet Forceps

Wrigley's forceps are used exclusively in outlet forceps operation.

Perineal and vulval infiltration with lignocaine is enough for local anesthesia.

Mid Forceps Operation

The most common indication for this is the manual rotation of the head, i.e. in malrotated occipitoposterior positon. The commonly used forceps is the long curved forceps with or without axis traction device.

Kielland's Forceps

It can be used in unrotated vertex or face presentation facilitating grasping and correction of a asynclitic head because of its sliding lock.

Difficulties in forceps operation

- Difficulty in locking
- Difficulty in traction
- Slipping of the blades.

Dangers of forceps operation

Maternal

Immediate complications are:

- Injury-laceration, cervical tear, perineal tear
- Nerve injury-femoral and lumbosacral
- Postpartum hemorrhage
- Anaesthetic complications
- Puerperal sepsis and maternal morbidity.

Remote

- Painful perineal scar
- Dyspareunia
- Low backache
- Genital prolapsed
- Sphincter dysfunction.

Fetal

Immediate

- Asphyxia
- Facial bruising

- Intracranial hemorrhage
- Cephalohematoma
- Facial palsy
- Skull fractures
- Cervical spine injury

Remote
- Cerebral/spastic palsy due to residual brain injury.

Ventouse or Vacuum Extractor

The vacuum extractor was introduced by Malmstorm. It is designed to apply traction to a cup attached to the fetal scalp. It allows the extraction and delivery of the fetal head in situations wherein the use of the obstetric forceps would be difficult or likely to be traumatic.

The vacuum extractor is an instrument designed to assist in delivery by creating a vacuum between its cups and the fetal scalp.

The instrument consists of a cup which is made to adhere to the fetal head by means of vacuum by creating negative pressure. The apparatus consists of ball shaped steel suction cups or silastic cups of 20 mm, 30 mm, 40 mm, 50 mm and 60 mm size, a traction chain covered by rubber tubing, a traction bar, a suction tubing made of rubber connecting the traction bar to the suction apparatus. A suction tubing made of rubber connecting the traction bar to the suction apparatus which creates a negative pressure by removing air or a separate opening for attachment of suction tubing. A manometer which is connected to the suction apparatus for pressure recordings.

Uses: It is an alternative to the obstetric forceps in the second stage of labor with the cervix fully dilated and the head low in the pelvis.

  i. In the first stage of labor, it can be of help as soon as the cervix is dilated enough to allow safe application of the cups if there are ineffective uterine contraction or malrotation.
  ii. It can be used along with the symphysiotomy in mild to moderate cases of disproportion.

Disadvantages

  i. Delivery may take longer.
 ii. The vacuum cup may become dislodged.
iii. Injuries to the maternal tissues are rare as compared to obstetric forceps.
 iv. Cannot help in case of fetal distress unlike the obstetric forceps as it needs time for Chignon to form.
  v. Cephalohematoma, intracranial injuries and necrosis of fetal scalp may result.
 vi. Can be used only in vertex presentations but cannot be used in premature babies.

Proposed classification: Proposed classification for vacuum extraction procedures according to fetal station and cranial position (ACOG 2000).

1. Outlet vacuum
Criteria
• Fetal head at or on perineum
• Scalp visible at introitus without separating labia
• Fetal skull has reached pelvic floor

2. Low vacuum
Criteria
• Criteria for outlet vacuum not fulfilled
• Leading edge of skull not reached pelvic floor
• Fetal skull not reached pelvic floor

Contraindications to use of Vacuum for Operative Vaginal Delivery

• Cephalopelvic disproportion
• Fetal head not engaged
• Gestational age is less than 34 weeks
• Known fetal conditions that affect bone mineralization or bleeding disorder
• Non-cephalic or facial presentation

Bibliography

1. Das S K, Mittal P, Suri S, Sinha R (200). Practical Manual of Obstetrics and Gynaecology: Instruments and Procedures (1st ed.): CBS Publishers and Distributors Pvt. Ltd.

2. Bennett VR, Brown LK (1996). Myles Textbook for Midwives (12th ed.). Edinburgh, London, Madrid, Melbourne, New York and Tokyo: Churchill Livingstone.

3. Bobak IM, Jensen MD, Lowdermilk DL (1989). Maternity and Gynecologic Care: (5th ed.): St. Louis Baltimore Boston Chicago London Philadelphia Sydney Toronto: Mosby.

4. Danforth et al. (2008). Danforth's Obstetrics and Gynecology (10th ed.): Philadelphia: Lippincott Williams and Wilkins.

5. Dutta DC (2015). Textbook of Obstetrics (8th ed.): The Health Sciences Publishers: New Delhi.

6. London ML, Ladewig. PW, Ball JW, Bindler RC (2011). Maternal and Child Nursing care (3rd ed.). New Jersey: Pearson Education, INC, Upper saddle river.

7. Pilitteri, A (1997). Maternal and Child Health Nursing: Care of the childbearing and childrearing family (7th ed.). Phildelphia: Lippincott Williams And Wilkins.

8. Reeder, Martin, Griffin K (1997). Maternity Nursing: Family, Newborn and Women's Health Care (18th ed.). Philadelphia: Lippincott.

9. Daftary SN. Chakravarthi, S (2011). Manual of Obstetrics (3rd ed.). New Delhi; Elsevier.

11 Destructive Operations and Instruments

Modern obstetrics is a field that is progressing rapidly. In the developed world, neglected labor is rarity; however, obstructed labor remains a reality. Most of the obstetricians resort to caesarean section deemed as the safest route of delivery. Moreover, expecting couples also prefer to have an elective cesarean section even in the absence of any indication. A critical concern in the field of obstetrics, however, is the management of obstructed labor when there is a dead fetus presentation. In this case, fetal destructive operations are chosen as on option, if the vaginal delivery is prolonged or obstructed. Destructive operations though do not have a place in modern obstetrics they are still considered as best options in low-resource settings wherein even if they are destructive, they are constructive for the mother.

What are destructive operations?

Destructive operations are designed to diminish the bulk of a dead fetus, i.e. reducing the size of the head, shoulder girdle or the whole body of the fetus to facilitate easy delivery per vaginum. The synonym of destructive operation is 'Embryotomy'.

What are the indications of destructive operations?

1. Patients having prolonged or obstructed labor with a dead fetus.
2. Hydrocephalus in a dead fetus where a simple perforation is enough.
3. Impacted fore-coming head as well as after-coming head of a dead fetus.

4. Delivery of grossly abnormal fetuses and congenital malformations, e.g. bicephalic monster.
5. Delivery of dead locked twins.

What are the absolute contraindications of destructive operations?

1. Live fetus
2. True conjugate less than 5.5 cm
3. Insuperable obstruction to vaginal delivery
4. Cervix less than three-fourths dilated and effaced
5. Threatened rupture of the uterus.

Types of destructive operations

1. Craniotomy
2. Evisceration
3. Decapitation
4. Cleidotomy

Craniotomy

An operation to make a perforation on the fetal head to evacuate the contents followed by the extraction of the fetus usually done with the help of a perforator.

Indications of craniotomy

- Cephalic presentation producing obstructed labor with dead fetus
- Hydrocephalus even in a living fetus
- Interlocking head of twins

Destructive instruments used for performing craniotomy

1. Perforators

Perforators are instruments used to perforate the skull of the dead fetus in order to reduce the bulk of the skull.

Sites of perforation performed in craniotomy

1. Vertex: Parietal bone (either side of the sagittal suture)
2. Face: Eye sockets/roof of mouth or through the orbit or hard palate
3. Brow: Frontal bone
4. Deflexed head: Dependent portion
5. After-coming head of breech presentation: Occiput, posterolateral fontanels, hard palate through the floor of mouth

Types of perforators
1.1. The Simpson's perforator

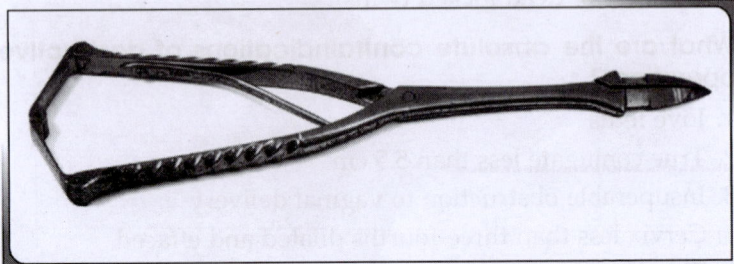

Fig. 11.1: The Simpson's perforator

1.2. Oldham's perforator

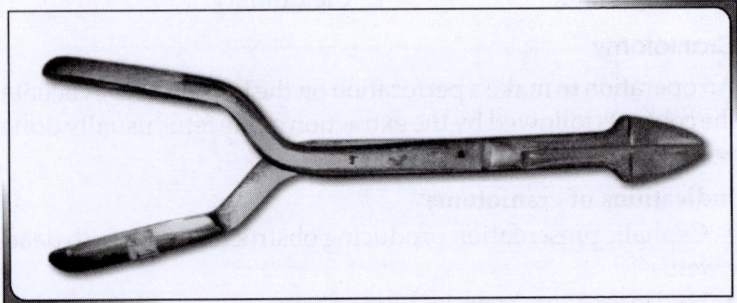

Fig. 11.2: Oldham's perforator

1.3. Smellie's perforator

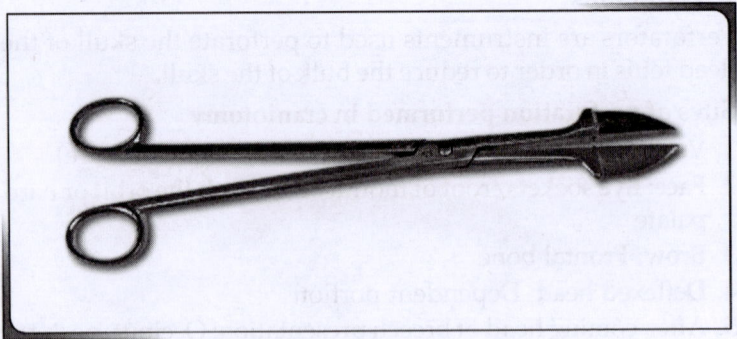

Fig. 11.3: Smellie's perforator

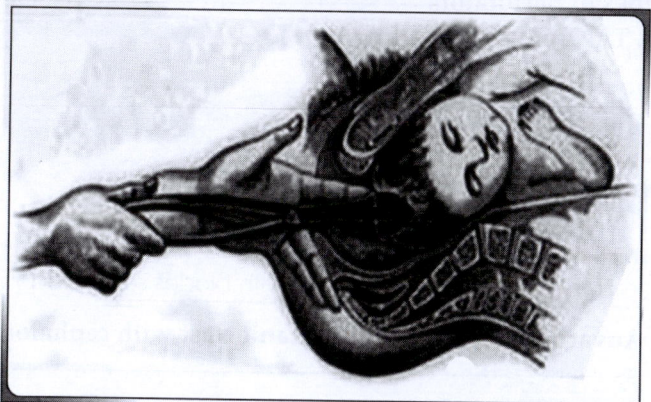

Fig. 11.4: Perforation performed using the Simpson's perforator on the vertex (site of the anterior fontanel) of the dead fetus

Uses of perforators: Perforators are employed to perforate the cranium in craniotomy. This is usually the first step involved in craniotomy.

2. Cranioclasts and Cephalotribes

Cranioclasts are destructive instruments that are akin to a very strong forceps, with which the skull of the dead fetus is crushed and then extracted per vaginum. Cephalotribes are destructive instruments, which also aid in crushing the skull of the dead fetus.

Types of Cranioclasts
2.1. Braun's Cranioclast

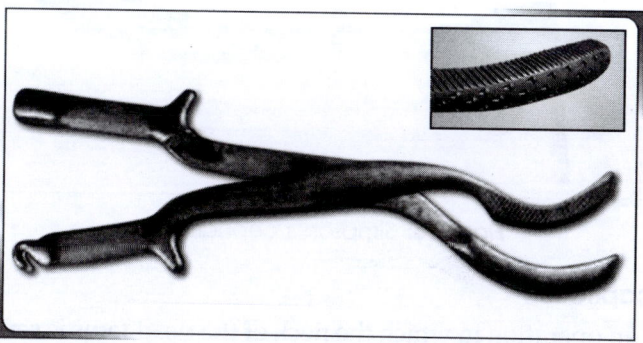

Fig. 11.5: Braun's cranioclast assembled

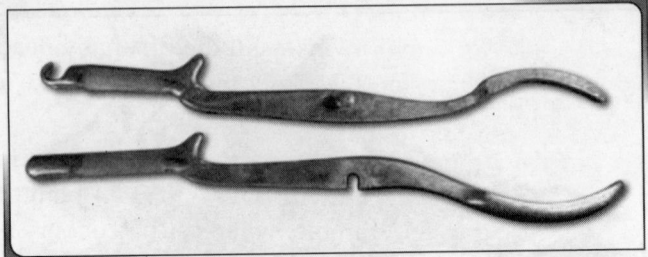

Fig. 11.6: Braun's cranioclast with blades separated

2.2. Auvard-Zweifel combined cranioclast with cephalotribe

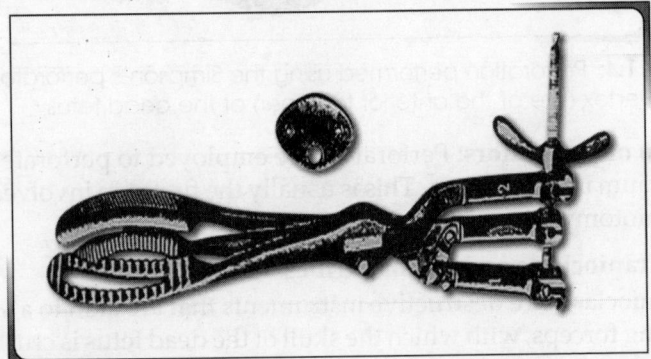

Fig. 11.7: Auvard-Zweifel combined cranioclast with cephalotribe

2.3. Simpson's cephalotribe

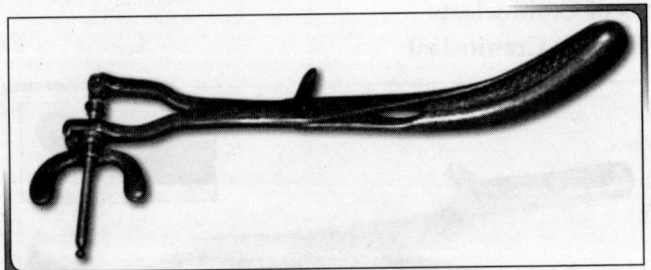

Fig. 11.8: Simpson's cephalotribe

Decapitation

It is an operation in which the neck of the dead fetus is severed from its trunk.

Indications of decapitation
- Impacted/neglected shoulder presentation with fetal neck accessible per vaginum
- Head to head locking of twins, with the first baby dead
- Double headed monster/Bicephalic monster in an obstructed labor

Destructive instruments used for performing decapitation
1. **Blonde-Heidler saw:** The wire saw is passed behind the foetal head using the thimble, whereas the rubber sheath covering the saw, protects the structures of the maternal birth canal. The detachable handles are then attached to both ends and the blade is pulled through the fetal neck, severing the neck in the process.

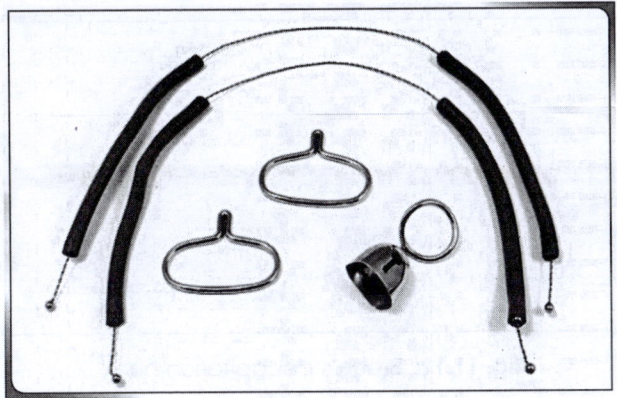

Fig. 11.9: Blonde-Heidler saw

2. **Dubois' embryotomy scissors**

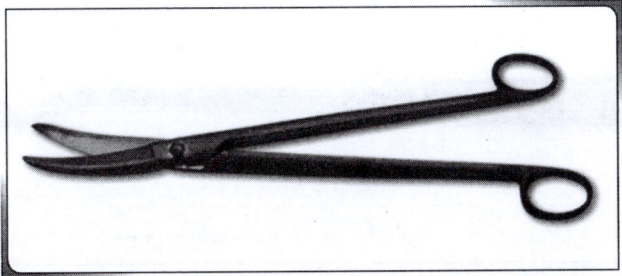

Fig. 11.10: Dubois' embryotomy scissors

3. Ramsbotham's decapitation knife

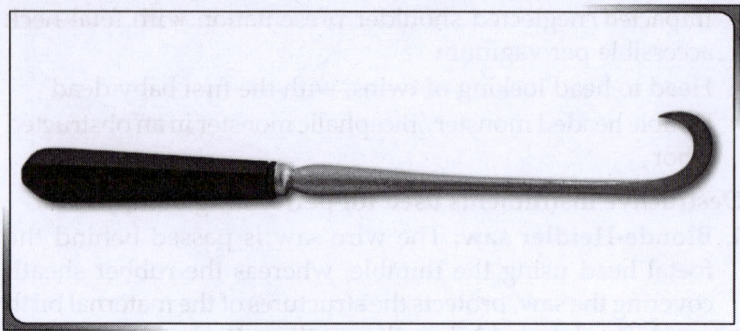

Fig. 11.11: Ramsbotham's decapitation knife

4. Braun's decapitation hook

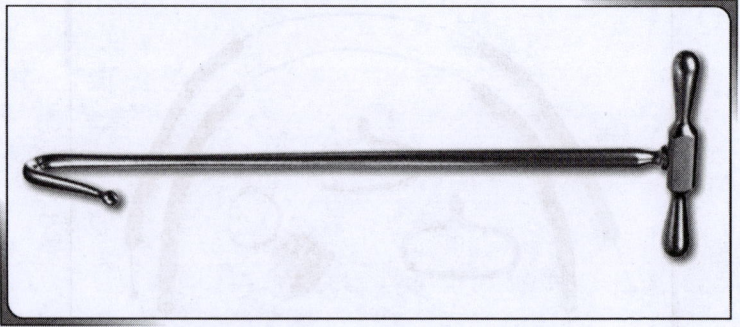

Fig. 11.12: Braun's decapitation hook

5. Jardine's decapitation hook

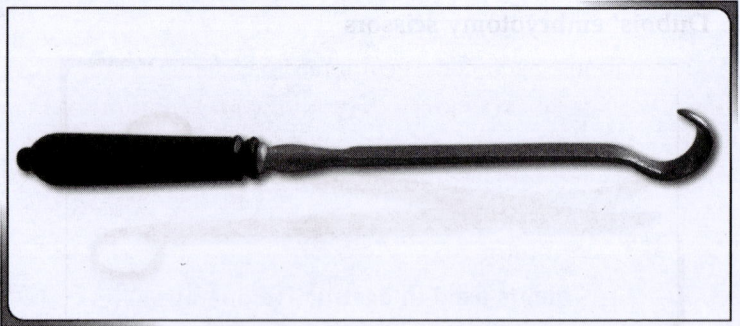

Fig. 11.13: Jardine's decapitation hook

6. Oldham's vertebral hook

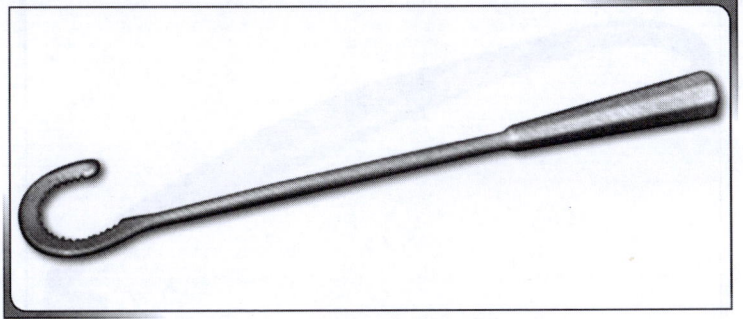

Fig. 11.14: Oldham's vertebral hook

Cleidotomy

Is an operation in which one or both the clavicles of the fetus are divided into two or more pieces. It reduces the bulk of the shoulder girdle by division of one or both the clavicles.

Indications for cleidotomy
- Shoulder dystocia
- Method failure

Evisceration

Operation in which the fetal thorax or the abdomen is opened and viscera of the fetus are removed piecemeal.

Indications for evisceration
- Fetal ascitis/hugely distended bladder of the dead fetus
- Monster
- Abdominal tumours
- Malformations: Sacrococcygeal teratoma, monstrosity
- Impacted shoulder/neglected shoulder presentation with dead fetus

Instruments used for cleidotomy and evisceration
1. Blunt hook and crochet
2. Hook with perforator

Ancillary instruments used in destructive operations
1. Blunt flushing curette
2. Bozeman's cannula

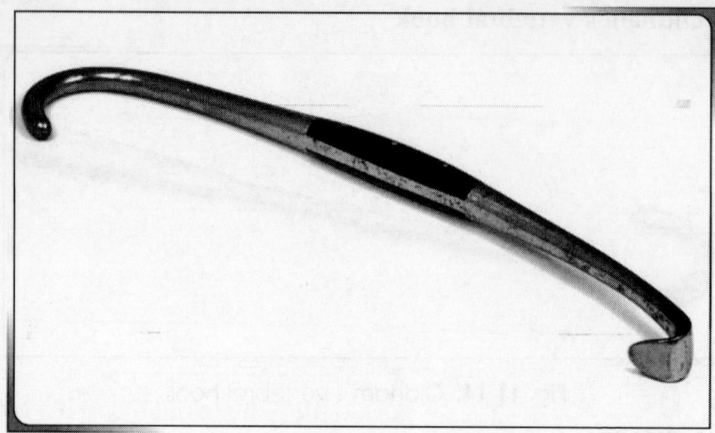

Fig. 11.15: Blunt hook and crochet

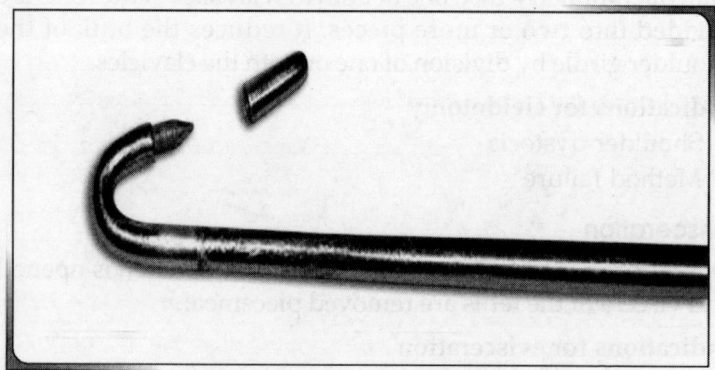

Fig. 11.16: Hook with perforator

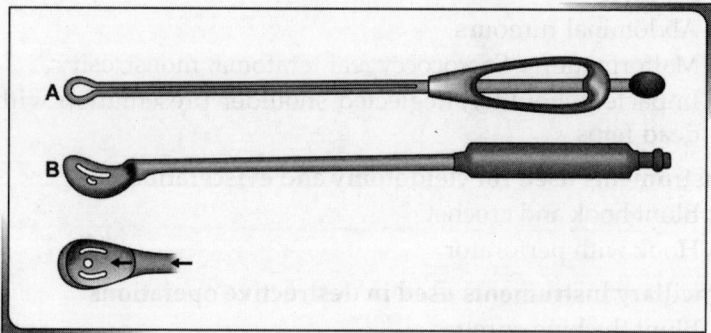

Fig. 11.17: Blunt flushing curette

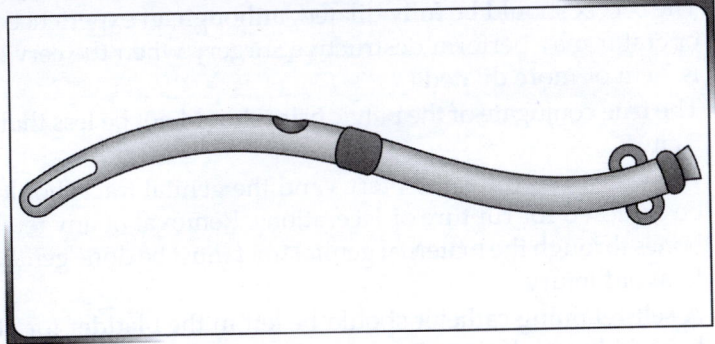

Fig. 11.18: Bozeman's cannula

Indications for using the ancillary instruments in destructive operations

1. To wash out the broken contents of fetal skull after craniotomy
2. Atonic postpartum hemorrhage: For intrauterine douche with antiseptic solution
3. Drainage of lochiometra

Midwives' role in conduct of destructive operations

Midwives are still the vital force in modern obstetrics, especially in low resource settings. It is pertinent that midwives are aware regarding the destructive operations used in obstetrics and the destructive instruments used.

Principles of Management

Important principles of management in the mother would be to correct the shock, dehydration, electrolyte deficit and acidosis.

- Hypovolemic shock may require infusion of crystalloids or colloids and blood transfusion using a central venous pressure manometer and urine output to monitor the fluid status.
- Broad-spectrum antibiotics are prescribed as septicemic shock may supervene at any stage.
- General anesthesia or regional anesthesia combined with sedation is ideal for the procedure.
- The abdomen should be examined for signs of uterine rupture or impending rupture and if present, a laparotomy is indicated, even if the fetus is dead.

- The cervix should be fully dilated, although an experienced operator may perform destructive surgery when the cervix is 7 cm or more dilated.
- The true conjugate of the pelvic brim should not be less than 8 cm.
- After the procedure, the uterus and the genital tract should be explored for rupture or lacerations. Removal of any fetal bones through the maternal genital tract must be done gently to avoid injury.
- A self-retaining catheter should be left in the bladder for at least 48 hours. If there has been prolonged pressure of the presenting part on pelvic structures, there is danger of fistula formation and the catheter should be left in the bladder for 10–14 days.
- Postpartum hemorrhage resulting from an atonic uterus should be avoided by commencing an infusion of 20–40 units of oxytocin immediately following the delivery of the baby. The patient should be nursed in a high-care setting or in a labor ward until stable.

Prerequisites for destructive operations

1. Patient should be given antibacterial drug therapy.
2. Preferably, two units of compatible blood should be kept ready to compensate for blood loss.
3. Secure an 18 G cannula IV line.
4. Ensure that cervix is preferable fully dilated and membranes are ruptured.
5. Prepared for general anesthesia; if need arises.

Postoperative care following destructive operations

1. Exploration of the uterovaginal canal to exclude rupture of the uterus or lacerations of vagina or any genital injury.
2. Foley's catheter is placed till the bladder tone is regained for a period of 3–5 days.
3. Dextrose saline drip continued till dehydration corrected
4. Ceftriaxone 1 g IV infusion twice daily

Complications of destructive operations

1. Injury to the uterovaginal canal: Maternal soft tissue trauma, i.e. vaginal, visceral, rectal trauma.

2. Rupture of uterus
3. Postpartum hemorrhage—atonic or traumatic
4. Shock due to blood loss or dehydration
5. Puerperal sepsis
6. Subinvolution
7. Injury to the adjacent viscera
8. Vesicovaginal fistula and rectovaginal fistula
9. Prolonged ill health.

Bibliography

1. Amo-Mensaha S, Elkins TE, Ghosh TS, Greenway CF, and Waite CV (1996). Brief communication—Obstetric destructive procedures. International Journal of Gynecology and Obstetrics. 54, 167–168.

2. Dutta DC. Destructive Operation in obstructed labour (1978). Journal of Indian Medical Association 72 (9).

3. Maharaj D, Moodley J. Symphysiotomy and fetal destructive operations. Best Practice and Research—Clinical Obstetrics and Gynaecology (2002). 16(1), 117–131.

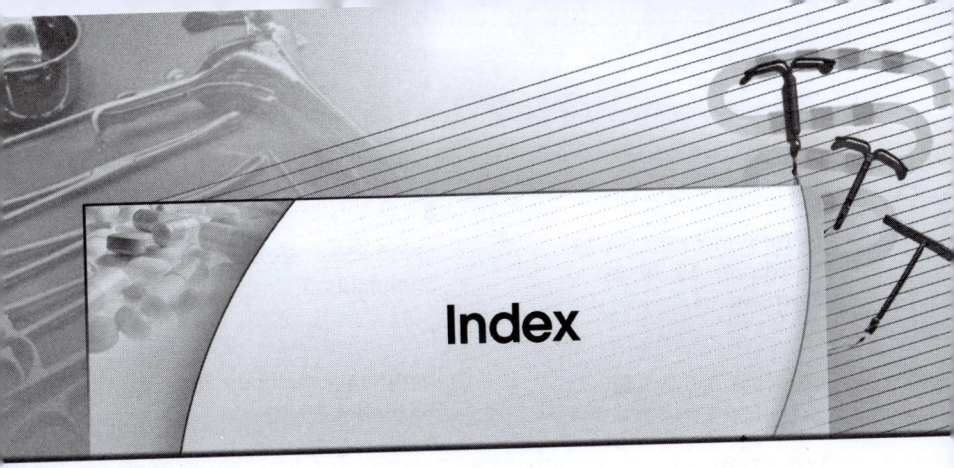

Index